EAT LIKE A PIG,
RUN LIKE A HORSE

EAT LIKE A PIG, RUN LIKE A HORSE

HOW FOOD FIGHTS HIJACKED OUR HEALTH

AND THE NEW SCIENCE OF EXERCISE

ANASTACIA
MARX DE SALCEDO

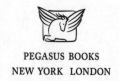

PEGASUS BOOKS

NEW YORK LONDON

EAT LIKE A PIG, RUN LIKE A HORSE

Pegasus Books, Ltd.
148 West 37th Street, 13th Floor
New York, NY 10018

First Pegasus Books cloth edition July 2022

Interior design by Maria Fernandez

ISBN: 978-1-64313-835-0

10 9 8 7 6 5 4 3 2 1

Printed in the United States of America
Distributed by Simon & Schuster
www.pegasusbooks.com

To the animals, who help us see

Chants Democratic

18.

Me imperturbe,
Me standing at ease in Nature,
Master of all, or mistress of all—aplomb in the
    midst of irrational things,
Imbued as they—passive, receptive, silent as they,
Finding my occupation, poverty, notoriety, foibles,
crimes, less important than I thought;
Me private, or public, or menial, or solitary—all
    these subordinate, (I am eternally equal with
    the best—I am not subordinate;)
Me toward the Mexican Sea, or in the Mannahatta,
    or the Tennessee, or far north, or inland,
A river-man, or a man of the woods, or of any farm-
    life of These States, or of the coast, or the lakes,
    or Kanada,
Me, wherever my life is lived, O to be self-balanced
    for contingencies!
O to confront night, storms, hunger, ridicule,
    accidents, rebuffs, as the trees and animals do.

—Walt Whitman, *Leaves of Grass*

Contents

Foreword

Being physically active is good for all ages. Allowing young kids to be physically active can set their habit of lifelong exercise. Being physically active in youth and as an adult reduces your risk of having any of the more than forty chronic diseases, for example, heart attacks, some cancers, type 2 diabetes, and others. Delaying chronic diseases lengthens your healthspan (the length of life before your first chronic disease). Also, being physically active could delay or even keep you out of a wheelchair in a nursing home. Finally, it reduces your chances of being depressed, making your life happier.

—Frank W. Booth, PhD,
Professor, University of Missouri

Preface

Last November, on a Staples run for office and school supplies, I pulled into the parking lot and immediately noticed a small flock of Canada geese standing in the middle of traffic, honking, all heads turned to the roof of the box store. I looked up. Pattering along the edge of the building was a fledgling. She teetered on the cornice, then picked her way west. The group, heedless of the jostle of cars in the access road, waddled after her, calling anxiously. I jumped out of my minivan and walked amid them, planting myself like a large CAUTION sign in the stream of vehicles. The fledgling halted at the far end of the roof. The geese cried in unison: "Come! Just flap your wings!" She strolled back to her original spot, but didn't move. Neither did I. I felt their heartbreak as keenly as if it were my own. I pictured them migrating together, the V formation alighting on top of the mall, and afterward, the young bird, for whatever reason—injury, fatigue, or fear, unable to continue. Eventually, I left. (Although I'd briefly fantasized about insisting that the Staples manager let me out on their roof.) But the image haunted me for the rest of the day and beyond. Did they save her?

When I first began this book, I decided to look at human metabolism, health, and disease through the lens of animals as a way to find a new perspective on a topic that has been examined innumerable times from an anthropocentric one. I think this approach allowed me to have fresh insights and make new linkages, but as time went on, it did something bigger: it made me feel more aware of animals and our relationship with them. On the other end of three-hundred-odd pages, I find myself quickly and utterly absorbed in watching two butterflies dance through cedar branches—why do they move that way and together?—or a bee crawling over a tiny pile of dirt into a hole in a railroad beam—what is she doing and where is she going?—and pulling to the curb to let my youngest daughter, Mariela, rescue a bunny that has become paralyzed with fear in the middle of the street. I hope some of the stories in this book will make you appreciate our fellow inhabitants of Planet Earth (even) more, especially ones, such as parasitic worms and bats, that often don't get a lot of human love.

When I describe *Eat Like a Pig, Run Like a Horse* to people, I often call it a crazy mix of personal narrative (many of the names and some details in these sections have been changed to protect privacy), journalism, and very easygoing science writing. There are reasons for all three of these things. I hope that knowing who I am, why I'm interested in things, and the connections I make between them encourages you to accompany me on my journey. This is also a feminist decision, since it is the opposite of the authoritative and disembodied third person, a distancing tradition that is sometimes used to cloak the (male) writer's intentions and (patriarchal) power. I have fully indulged my aversion to quotations that are just a couple of phrases or sentences. The reason? I like people to speak for themselves. Before interviews, I brief myself thoroughly on their background and topic, so our conversation is about their particular expertise. My job is to be the conduit; quoting long passages allows each of these fascinating people to present themselves and their ideas directly to you. And finally, to make the science comprehensible to everyone, I've kept those sections extremely simple and in layperson's language. If you want to reconstruct my (extensive) research, all sources are listed in the bibliography. I am also happy to explain the concepts and arguments in more detail—just write.

No book introduction would be complete without acknowledgments. I am blessed to have both an amazing editor and agent who wholeheartedly supported my creativity and experimentation. Thank you so much, Jessica Case and Stephany Evans, for taking risks with me. I'm appreciative of the busy scientists—Laurie Goodyear, Darrell Neufer, and Michael Sturek—who took the time to review some of my science passages. Jessica LeTourneur Bax braved my misuse of hyphens and dashes and gently corrected some descriptions and terms. Derek Thornton enriched the book with a semaphoric cover and Maria Fernandez, with comfy interior pages. I am also very grateful for the encouragement and friendship of my writing buddy, Rebecca Lemov. Finally, thank you to my family for tolerating having some of our most intimate moments made public and for making every one of my days an adventure.

1

Poster Child for Multiple Sclerosis

On a sunny, spring day in April 1991, I woke up in the South End railroad apartment I shared with my boyfriend of five years—inseparable since Columbia College—fretting about work. Should I check one more time with the Boat and Recreation Vehicle Registration and Titling Bureau to see if they had the total number of 1990 boat licenses yet? Not having the latest year's information would make my report look outdated before it had even been printed. But if they did, I'd have to do a whole new economic impact analysis.

Our coffeemaker gave a final gurgle in the kitchen, and then Mack appeared with two steaming cups. He set his on the bureau as he dressed: button-down shirt, brown chinos, sweater. Our brick building—most distinguishing feature, a faded 1960s-era, black-and-yellow fallout shelter sign—was a forty-five-minute walk and subway ride from the Harvard University Department of Mathematics where he was writing a computer program to model Riemann surfaces for a professor.

"Working from home again?" Mack asked, sipping his coffee. For the past couple weeks, I'd been holed up in our apartment writing a strategic plan for the Massachusetts maritime industry, a project I was doing for my research support staff job at Harvard Business School.

"I concentrate better here. No interruptions," I smiled, shaking my hand vigorously, as if it were on fire and I was trying to put it out.

"What are you doing?"

"Slept on it wrong. It's asleep." According to my mother, Ida Petroni, the Italian grandmother who lived downstairs from us in the apartment I was born in, on Second Avenue and 116th Street in Manhattan, insisted I should be forced to sleep on my back as a newborn. This may have precipitated a lifetime of authority issues: unless I am facedown, X-sprawled, and drooling, I wake up in a panic. Sometimes I crush my bent hands beneath my torso, so I occasionally wake up with pins and needles in my fingers.

"Mmm." Mack went to shave and brush his teeth in the bathroom at the other end of the apartment. I flexed and straightened the fingers on my right hand. At least ten minutes had gone by since I'd woken up and still no feeling. Odd.

By midmorning, my hand was still numb. I called Mack.

"I think I've got carpal tunnel or something," I told him. It made perfect sense. I was now on my second book-length project at the research center. Over the three years since I'd graduated, I'd typed up the notes from hundreds of interviews, written dozens of memos, and cranked out two manuscripts. I tended to pound my keyboard, which, at Harvard Business School, was on my desk, forcing my arms into an awkward, crooked position. Here at home, I had a special computer hutch—designed solely for all the bulky components of the original personal computers. A sliding tray underneath housed the keyboard, but I still banged as if it were a rusty, old typewriter from the 1920s. I wrapped an Ace bandage around my right wrist and didn't give it much more thought.

When I woke up the next morning, there was a lidded mug of coffee on my nightstand. Mack had already left. We'd bought it as a set of two in Chinatown during one of our many meandering walks through New York City a few years before. The black ceramic was covered with a lattice of delicate flowers; the sight made me happy, as did the anticipation of the hot, bitter liquid. I reached out my arm. But I couldn't lift it. My bicep felt shaky and weak; my fingers wouldn't close around the handle. I sat up in bed, throwing back the green-and-beige, bear-claw-pattern cover and swinging my legs over the side. I stood. My right thigh tingled and felt unstable, as if it would buckle under my weight.

What was wrong with me?

I called my health maintenance organization's urgent care line. My physician immediately referred me to a neurologist. I then called my parents, who lived nearby, and asked if they could take me to the appointment. An hour or so later, their white Toyota Camry inched down our street. That my mother had driven alone to Boston was a testament to the gravity of the situation. In her twenties, she'd day-dreamed through a stop sign and been hit from both sides by oncoming cars. She'd refused to drive for over a decade, and after that, only to the grocery store one mile from our house. I maneuvered my way out of the first-floor apartment like an old person: bracing myself on furniture, clinging to doorframes and handles, lowering myself cautiously down the granite front steps. Once in the car, I leaned my head back on the seat. I was exhausted.

The neurology department was at the Kenmore Center, which had its own parking garage. But the five-story building was big and spread out, and with each step, the distances to the garage elevator, to the admissions desk, and then up to the fourth floor and to the office, located at the very end of a long set of hallways, seemed to grow. I could barely pull myself across the navy blue carpets. Even my mother, who lugged 180 pounds on her 5'4" frame and was already pinched by osteoarthritis, outpaced me. Once there, we sat in a tiny waiting room. I looked around nervously. What lay in store for me? A father and daughter flanked a crying middle-aged woman, her husband rubbing her back. Another woman, her face gray and drawn, flicked uninterestedly through a magazine. A man with black hair and thick glasses buzzed by in a wheelchair.

"Dr. Grim will see you now." A physician's assistant escorted me to an examination room, weighed—128 pounds—and measured—5'5"—me. She took my blood pressure, which was normal. After a while, Dr. Grim entered the room and brusquely pulled up a stool. "You're experiencing numbness and weakness on one side? Since when?" he asked urgently. "What was the first symptom?" He took out a little hammer with a triangular, rubber head and tapped me below each knee. He pricked the bottoms of my feet and along the skin of my shins and forearms with a needle. "Push down!" he commanded, inserting his hands under my palms. "Now up," he said, turning them over and covering them with his black-haired hand. He took out a small penlight and asked me to follow it with my eyes. Then he had me walk back and forth in a straight line across the floor.

"I think we can rule out a stroke," he said. "Not only highly unlikely at your age, but you don't have any other symptoms. Which leaves three possibilities." He didn't smile, and he didn't look me in the eye; instead he scribbled on his pad. "It's possible it's an anomaly. After a few weeks, you'll get better, and that will be that. It could be a brain tumor, in which case you may experience a worsening of symptoms. If this happens, you'll need to come back. We'll schedule you for a CT scan [this was just before MRIs became common], and if there is a mass, biopsy it. And finally, it could be multiple sclerosis. In which case, this would be the first of many episodes, and will eventually lead to disability and a shortened life span." He swiveled in his chair. "Here's a pamphlet. Any questions?"

Questions? Where to begin? But I said nothing. I was twenty-seven. When this began, I'd woken up sweating a detail of a hundred-page report. Now my future, solid, safe, and dull—apply to grad school (economics maybe?), marry Mack, write and paint when I could, kids?—had suddenly evaporated. In its place was the vulnerability and uncertainty of illness. I was terrified.

So I did what any sane person would have done in my circumstances: I fled.

∞

Three years later, in February 1994, I woke up in the sun-flooded Quito, Ecuador, apart-suite (the South American version of single-room occupancy housing) I shared with my boyfriend, Rafael, to find him standing next to the bed. He was wearing the black-and-white kimono bathrobe I'd spotted in a Goodwill store and immediately known was for him and holding a steaming cup of coffee. "Burrita" ("little donkey," his nickname for me; long story), he said, "cafecito." I extended my hand for the mug, decorated with a gaily colored *chiva*, the open-air buses used in rural Colombia, but my fingers just brushed clumsily over the handle and refused to close. My left hand had gone numb. From there, everything happened just as it had before, except on the opposite side of my body: gripping sensations over my abdomen, a foot I couldn't feel or lift, extreme fatigue. (The symptoms from my first attack had long since disappeared, except for a tiny numb spot on my right thumb, like an annoying neurological hangnail.)

In the past three years, I had remade myself. I no longer worked at Harvard Business School nor planned a career in academia. I'd moved to South America, living there by myself, and started a successful business, an English-language newspaper. I'd first drifted apart from and then broken up with Mack. It was amicable. We still loved each other, and we both believed that we'd somehow continue. But in the meantime, I'd fallen into a tempestuous affair with a Cuban journalist. And I was different: bold, confident, and unafraid.

After my visit with Dr. Grim, I had frozen in fear. All I could think about were canes and wheelchairs, of not being able to feel a caress, of seeing double or not at all, of losing control of my bladder and bowels, of not being able to get aroused or have an orgasm. I was constantly surveying my body, braced against the onset of my next attack. Was that tingle in my foot normal? That temporary darkening of my vision?

A moment of midmorning lightheadedness (maybe skipping breakfast wasn't such a great idea?). It was draining. After several months, out of simple self-preservation, I pushed those images to the deepest recesses of my mind.

I began exercising again as soon as I could. During the weeks after my attack, I'd returned to the pool—I had been swimming a mile five days a week—with ferocious intensity. My tingling arm and leg felt like arcs of sparkles as they cut into the water, but I finished every workout. In the spring, Mack and I began taking long bike rides around the working-class coastal towns and neighborhoods that surround Boston like a collar: South Boston, Charlestown, East Boston, Chelsea, Everett, Winthrop, Revere. My limbs regained feeling and strength, which made the brain tumor unlikely. So either I'd lucked out and this was an anomaly, never to recur and relegated to a scary story told at long, boozy dinner parties, or I had multiple sclerosis, undecipherable, incurable, and untreatable (then, before interferon-based therapies had been discovered).

Mack applied to graduate school to study chaos theory and decided to attend Stanford. My plan was to go with him and fulfill my dream of becoming a writer. But first we would travel by land from the United States to South America. Destination: São Paulo, Brazil, where Mack had been an exchange student when he was sixteen. We started in San Diego, descending by bus through Mexico, Guatemala, Honduras, Nicaragua, and Costa Rica. We decided to skip hiking the Darién Gap, the sixty-six-mile break in the Pan-American Highway between Panama and Colombia, and flew directly to Ecuador, to meet Mack's older sister, Sue.

After spending a couple weeks with her there, Mack and I flew to Cali, Colombia. Mack, who was the best gift-giver I've ever known, had arranged one of my all-time favorite days, tagging along in a jeep with an agricultural program manager in Armenia, the country's coffee production center, as he visited large haciendas and small fincas to check on crops and livestock. Then we continued north to the Lost City (accessible only by a week's trek through the jungle), Santa Marta, and finally Cartagena. We walked around in the sultry heat, holding hands, goggling at the colonial architecture and gorgeous tropical colors, eating Colombian food and drinking wine, and wandering into musical venues from jazz and salsa to traditional *vallenatos*.

The next day, we took the bus to the Rafael Núñoz International Airport. It was August 1992, and Mack's mathematics program began in a few days. At the international terminal, we hugged each other tightly. "See you soon. I love you," I said, and he boarded his American Airlines flight to San Francisco. Holding back tears, I stumbled onto the shuttle to the domestic terminal and got in line for an Avianca flight to Bogotá, where I'd live for a month with a Colombian friend. Then, trying to make my $10,000 in savings last as long as they could, I took a bus back to Quito, Ecuador, where everything was cheaper. I'd been there ever since.

I wasn't about to lose my newfound sangfroid. I dressed, struggled down four flights of stairs, and limped to the bus stop on Avenida 6 de Diciembre. When it stopped—well, slowed—I grabbed the rail firmly and hauled myself aboard. I usually hopped off when we hit the touristy Mariscal neighborhood in Quito's "New City," full of nice restaurants and high-rises, and strode the seven or eight blocks to my one-room office on Calle Juan Léon Mera. Today I practically crept. No matter. I got there and sat down at my desk, a repurposed wooden table from a shuttered restaurant.

On hearing about my illness and the possible diagnoses, my partner, a socialist Chilean who'd fled after Pinochet's coup d'état, suggested we schedule a sales meeting with the neurology department of the Hospital de Clínicas Pichincha. Our small business generated just enough money to cover the wages of a second editor and a secretary and two extremely modest stipends for ourselves (sales and distribution staff were paid commissions). We offered a *canje*, a trade: a half-page ad for six months advertising their new, cutting-edge diagnostic tool, the MRI, in return for using it on one of the publishers. The medical center, salivating at the prospect of reaching Ecuador's cash-rich gringos and oil industry–affiliated expatriates, surprised us by saying yes.

Although they'd explained that it wouldn't hurt, I was nervous the day of the test. I put on a johnny and then lay down on a narrow, white table that slid in and out of what looked like the nose cone of a rocket. Inside, it was close and dark. I shut my eyes. A banging began. It went on for a while, then seemed to shift direction. Then again. Then it stopped. Then it resumed from a completely different angle. The whole exam took perhaps thirty to forty minutes. Afterward, I got dressed and went back to my day, assigning articles; troubleshooting obstacles with writers; editing; sending out bills by messenger; debriefing and encouraging salespeople as they made their rounds; overseeing Lilia, my Colombian secretary; and dealing with the constant stream of visitors—readers, writers, jobseekers—who passed by the office.

A few days later, Rafi and I returned to get the results. We sat in two chairs on the other side of the desk of the neurologist, a tall, curly-haired man. We exchanged extended pleasantries—no Ecuadorian interaction happens without them: where we were from, what we were doing, our Romeo (Cuba) and Juliet (the United States) romance.

"Bueno," the doctor said. "This is something I haven't seen before. There are many lesions on your brain." My breathing seemed to stop. "We have no cases of it here in Ecuador. But I saw some when I was a resident in Mexico City. I think it is multiple sclerosis." The bottom of my stomach fell to the floor. I began to cry. Rafi held my hand, although he, too, had no familiarity with the disease. But I did. And I knew what it meant. I may have run away, but death had tracked me down again.

I spent the next few days feeling very sorry for myself, alternately sobbing and sleeping on the lumpy, full-size mattress in our tiny suite, which consisted of a space just big enough for a bed and bureau, a small bathroom, and a narrow hall-like extension with a tiny glass table and two chairs. I meditated, trying to cure myself by channeling the force of the universe through a Y shape I imagined entering both sides of my brain. I'd visualize healing energy coursing through the loops, twists, and dead ends of tissue until I saw shimmers. Then I'd get down on the floor and do endless exercises: push-ups, sit-ups, leg lifts. Then I'd doze.

In the afternoon, as the light dimmed and shadow overtook our room, my optimism wilted. I categorized my impairments: numb and dragging left foot, an impression that something was crawling over my midriff, a hand that couldn't close around a pen. During the day, my editor had come by with some checks for me to sign. My writing resembled chicken scratches. By the time Rafi came home from his job as cultural editor of *La Hora*, a national tabloid, it was around 9:00 P.M., and I was in despair. He brought me some chicken and french fries, but I didn't want to eat. I wanted to have sex, to feel my body, to forget myself. We did, but when he entered me, it set off weird detonations in my thigh, my knee, the sole of my foot. Concentrating very hard, I came. And then I cried.

"What's going to happen to me? Am I going to be disabled? Will I need a wheelchair?"

"Will you marry me?" Rafi asked.

∾

I had the flu, but I put on charcoal wool pants, a pink wool turtleneck, and high, brown boots anyway. Since our daughter, Esmerelda, was born in fall 1996, I'd been cold-calling banks, hospitals, health centers, energy companies, nonprofits, and government agencies—anyone who might have a need for multilingual materials. It was now January 1998, and Rafi's and my small advertising business was finally taking off. But we couldn't afford to lose a single client.

A light snow tapped the windshield as I drove to Hyde Park High School, where Étienne Georges, our Haitian Creole translator, worked as a guidance counselor. "How is your daughter?" he asked. I asked about his son. I sat in the hard student chair in front of his desk while he reviewed the glossy proofs the printer had dropped on our front steps at 5:00 A.M. that morning. After Étienne, I would drive to Union Square to visit Vicente Lopes, a doctor, who worked at the Massachusetts Alliance of Portuguese Speakers and did our Cape Verdean translations. Every word of the brochure and poster for prenatal services—which we'd created in four different languages—needed to be perfect. If I approved the job to run by 5:00 P.M., it would be printed that night, cut and folded in the morning, and delivered to our client, a community health center, the next day.

When I got home, I was exhausted and shivering. I staggered into bed. The next day, when I woke up, my left leg felt cold, as if it had been left in an invisible refrigerator. When I stood, I wobbled. And there was an electrical sensation that stopped and started at regular intervals. After a week of laying low and coddling myself, the symptoms seemed to subside, and I returned to regular life. (Okay, regular life if that included my thighs and soles being repeatedly stabbed as I walked.)

I also made an appointment with a new neurologist. After my experience in Ecuador, my mother had begun to donate to multiple sclerosis research in my name, and every month, a thin magazine, *Inside MS*, slid through the mail slot. I never cracked the spine. Why learn about the depressing things that were happening to the other people with my disease? One day, my father, who worked as a consulting statistician in the pharmaceutical industry, called me very excited. The FDA had recently approved a new drug created by his employer. The clinical trials seemed to show that interferon, a signaling protein that blocks the messages that activate inflammation, slowed disease progression. "Would you think about taking it, honey?"

Dr. David Pilgrim smiled an awful lot for someone who spent his day dealing with neurology patients, whose disorders tend to range from the merely serious—stroke, Parkinson's, epilepsy, and MS—to full-on catastrophic—aneurysms, brain tumors, and amyotrophic lateral sclerosis (ALS). "So what's going on?" he asked, scooching his desk chair over to the table where I sat with long, narrow feet. As I told him, he rapidly went through the office neurological exam—hammer below the knees, push-pull, follow the light, walk, bend over.

"Let's get you an MRI. That should give us a clearer picture of what's causing this."

When I saw Dr. Pilgrim again, he pinned several black-and-white films up on a light board and gave me a tour of my brain. "See these foci, these white circles, here," he pointed to a spot close to one of the two dark ventricles on the top of the brain. "These are the plaques from your first attacks. They would have affected your motor ability and sensation on each side of your body. But what you're experiencing now, the weakness and paresthesia in your left leg, comes from a lesion on your spine. This one right here, down about the lumbar region. So, how are you feeling?"

"A lot better," I said. "I'm already swimming again. How soon can I go back to inline skating?" He laughed.

"Whenever you want. Don't you want to hear about some of the new drugs on the market for treating multiple sclerosis?"

"Not really. I've read up on them, and as far as I can see, they don't really offer much for me. My flare-ups are infrequent—every couple of years, and, until now, I've had complete recovery between them. When I weigh the possibility of further slowing an already slow progression against the discomfort of giving myself a shot that feels like a weekly case of the flu, the answer seems clear. But what do you think, Dr. Pilgrim?"

He smiled kindly. "I think you're right. And if things change for you later on, we can always revisit the decision. By the way," he added. "There's evidence that shows regular physical activity may be just as good as these new treatments in slowing disease progression. Where do you skate?"

"On Saturdays, I practice skills in the schoolyard near my house. And on Sundays, I like to go around the river. You have to look out for twigs, acorns, and big cracks, though, or you can end up flat on your . . . but there's nothing like skating outside in nature. It's like flying." It was how I felt right now, too. Validated. Respected. This intelligent man—one of the best doctors I've ever had—was frankly acknowledging the limits of medicine and supporting my decision to flaunt the conventional wisdom about how to treat my illness.

∽

And so it went.

Every few years, generally after some kind of viral infection— conjunctivitis, an upper respiratory illness—or a period of high stress and sleeplessness, I'd have a flare-up. Nothing like the first two attacks, which had been devastating. The bottom of my foot would go numb. Crawling sensations would wrap one or both thighs (these triggered what I dubbed "footgasms," jolts in my foot when I'm aroused or climaxing). The fatigue that's a fact of my daily life (the antidote: mugs of weapons-grade java) would become insurmountable, and I'd have to lie down. At first, there was always a moment of panic. Would this exacerbation be the one that permanently disabled me? The one that presaged a shift in the course of my disease from relapsing-remitting (up-and-down hills) to primary progressive (straight line down)?

I talked myself through these troughs. Relax. Take care of yourself. Trust your body. I'd rest, keeping the affected body part warm (somehow I didn't notice the symptoms as much that way). I'd redouble my self-care, doing my weird healing meditation with the inverted Y several times a day. I tried to sleep as much as I wanted—or at least as much as I was able to as the mother of young children and the owner of a small business.

As soon as the symptoms began to dissipate, I'd get up and drag myself around—this was sometimes literally true, as a leg might not be functioning normally. I had to concentrate extra hard when I drove. Once, when my right foot was numb and I couldn't feel the pressure of the gas pedal, I accidentally accelerated to ninety miles per hour on the highway. I'd pass people walking on the street and envy how they took their legs for granted. No one, not the chubby, middle-aged man plodding home from work; the slender runner high-stepping while he waited for the walk signal; or the irritated-looking mother grabbing at two toddlers as they balanced on the black-flecked granite curb, appreciated the marvel. But slowly, with advances and retreats, I'd get better.

And I always kept exercising.

I am now fifty-seven. I weigh 130–135 pounds. My blood pressure varies from 120/80 down to 100/60, depending on how agitated I am. My blood cholesterol is perfect, with a ratio of two and very low triglycerides. In fact, in the decades since my first MS attack, most of my ailments have been sports injuries.

∽

"What skin-care products do you use?" the medical assistant asked when I went for an urgent care appointment after spraining my ankle last summer. First time they'd ever asked me this question as part of taking my vital signs. Perhaps there was something I should be avoiding for some reason? Or a medication that they might prescribe for me that could be affected by something topical?

"Different things," I said. "But mostly natural ones. Kiss My Face vitamin A & E lotion for my body and Kiss My Face 50 SPF sunscreen for my face." The medical assistant wrote down the names on a piece of paper. "Why do they collect that information?"

"Oh, I'm asking for myself! Your skin is so beautiful, and you look, you know, like you are in your thirties!"

"The best thing for your skin is exercise," I said. "I run every day. I lift weights and dance. It makes me happy, gives me energy, and makes me look good—including my skin." She wasn't persuaded. "What's the exact name of the body lotion?"

When the doctor came in, she examined my ankle. It was as large as a baseball, and there was a stripe of purple about an inch above the outside of my sole. But I didn't cry out when she asked me to bend it left, right, up, and down. "I don't think anything's broken, but if you have more pain, you should call me, and we'll schedule an X-ray for you. Meanwhile, RICE. You know what that means, right? Rest, ice, compression, and elevation."

"Yes, I know," I said. "When can I go back to running? It's really important for me to exercise every day. I have MS, and it helps me keep exacerbations at bay."

"You have MS?" A look of shock cracked her professional veneer. Then she recovered. "You should stay off the ankle until it's completely healed, at least a couple of weeks."

I am a medical miracle.

∞

"How are you feeling?" Sue, Mack's older sister, asks me whenever we see each other. We'd remained friends after the breakup, and whenever she's here from the Netherlands—she'd become life partners with a Dutch dockworker and they have two children—we tried to work in a visit, either in New York, Boston, or at my family home in Vermont as she traveled to her other brother's home in Burlington. The question always made me wither inside. I knew it came from kindness, but her solicitude reminded me that most people with MS battle a catalog of health complaints. I didn't want to think about it, and I certainly didn't want it to be the first thing people thought about me.

Now, however, as I've become more confident in my disease's benign course, I've become more curious. After twenty-seven years, 93 percent of patients have disabilities, ranging from small impairments to being bedridden, according to a 2011 New York University School of Medicine analysis of the national MS registry.[1] At one of our appointments, Dr. Pilgrim laughingly called me the poster child for MS. At our last, at which he told me he was leaving the practice, I asked him if I should get a neurological checkup every couple of years. He shrugged. "Only if you want to," he told me. "Just keep on doing whatever it is you're doing."

But what was that? My diet? I eat a lot of vegetables, nuts, seeds, and plant oils. Starting in the 1950s, a low-fat, plant-based diet had been advocated to control MS by Roy Swank, a neurologist at the University of Oregon. Although the diet has its adherents to this day, it was soundly debunked in a 2016 randomized, controlled study led by Vijayshree Yadav, also a neurologist at the University of Oregon.[2] Getting regular sunshine? Some studies link the disease to the reduced solar vitamin D exposure further from the equator. The glass of wine I drink every night—and sometimes more on the weekends? There was nothing more regular in my life than physical activity—and my symptoms seemed to reappear quickly when I stopped. But if so, why did exercise have such a powerful protective effect—not only keeping me from getting run-of-the-mill lifestyle illnesses, but allowing me to coexist with one of humankind's twelve most debilitating diseases, according to *Healthcare Business & Technology*?

---

1   Ilya Kister et al., "Disability in Multiple Sclerosis: A Reference for Patients and Clinicians," *Neurology* 80, no. 11 (2013): 1018–24.

2   Vijayshree Yadav et al., "Low-Fat, Plant-Based Diet in Multiple Sclerosis: A Randomized Controlled Trial," *Multiple Sclerosis and Related Disorders* 9 (2016): 80–90.

I decided to find out. It turned out that our understanding of MS was evolving. It was no longer viewed as simply an autoimmune and inflammatory disorder, but, as I'd experienced firsthand, a disease with a strong metabolic component. Researchers had linked unhealthy lipid profiles—high LDL (bad cholesterol) and triglyceride levels—with increased and more severe MS exacerbations. Those with high HDL (good cholesterol), on the other hand, experienced fewer attacks.[3] Other scientists documented a protective effect with both alcohol (yay!) and physical activity.[4] We already know that exercise prevents and can treat heart disease, stroke, vascular disease, high blood pressure, high cholesterol, and diabetes. So you'd think that there would be a well-developed body of scientific research showing how. But shockingly, we know very little about how regular movement translates into changes at the cellular and molecular level. In the past decade and a half, that's begun to shift. This book describes my journey as I explore this new and life-altering science—and why it should radically change everyone's priorities for daily self-care.

---

3 Bianca Weinstock-Guttman et al., "Serum Lipid Profiles Are Associated with Disability and MRI Outcomes in Multiple Sclerosis," *Journal of Neuroinflammation* 8 (2011): 127.

4 Marie Beatrice D'Hooghe, Guy Nagels, Véronique Bissay, and Jaques De Keyser, "Modifiable Factors Influencing Relapses and Disability in Multiple Sclerosis," *Multiple Sclerosis: Clinical and Laboratory Research* 16, no. 7 (2010): 773–85.

2

Fat Cats and Diabetic Dogs

Ready?" Mariela, my youngest, then thirteen, asks me. I nod. Mariela cups Willy's taut belly. I cradle tiny Luna, her sage eyes alarmed. It is the moment of reckoning for our relationship with the kittens, both rescues, who we got about a month ago. Mariela butt-checks open the back door, I plow through, and we are out. We hustle across the deck, down the steps, and along the brick path to a small patio in the middle of the yard. After weeks of cold, wet weather, every single tree, bush, and flower is in bloom, as if spring had been turned on with a switch. Mariela and I position the baby cats in the lawn beside the patio. They are electrified. The grass! The trees! The sun! The breeze! Birds, butter-flies, insects, and squirrels! Will they come back when called? Willy charges up the dogwood trunk; Luna chases a bee. They run and jump, sniff, and nibble, drunk on the pleasure of being in nature. Mariela and I trail behind, detaching them from trunks and blocking them when their forays go beyond the ten-by-ten foot patch of green. After about twenty minutes, they return willingly to our arms, and we bring them inside. Their first outing has been a success.

From then on, we visit the yard on a regular basis, one human per kitten, like nervous toddler parents at the playground. At first, we limit the area to the side-by-side patio and square of grass. But as they get more familiar with their environment—and more reliable in returning to us, we let them roam more widely: into the tall redbud and cherry trees, along the gray, wooden fence that divides our plot of earth from the surrounding houses, and around the corner into the side garden bursting with rose bushes. Rafi builds a simulated litter box, dirt topped by a layer of kitty litter, to teach them how to do their business outside. As would any good cat mother, he demonstrates correct elimination hygiene, crouching, scuffling the dirt with his hands, hovering his rear over the hole, and then carefully filling it up. Eventually, when the kittens are in late adolescence, we permit them to spend an hour or so outside alone, calling them in by shaking the treat bag before they can get too far. They don't stray much anyway. By early autumn, when they are nine months or so, the pair go in and out at will, letting us know their wishes by standing at the back door—as befits two species cohabiting on an equal footing.

Their behavior out mirrors their behavior in. Willy, with apricot fur and one slightly protruding eyetooth, is expansive. Rescued with his litter, he has never known loneliness. Luna is his opposite: a meager shadow, found alone in the New England February cold. In their foster home, she'd glommed onto Willy and not let go. Luna startles at every loud noise and sudden movement, relying on Willy to mediate the world for her. Do they need food? Want to be let out? Willy fetches us from our basement offices, tip-toeing on his hind feet alongside our desk chairs, looking beseechingly at us, and tapping our legs with his paw (claws fully retracted). He is irresistible. "Okay, Willy," I sigh, and go upstairs to pour some dry food in their side-by-side feeder. Luna will only exit and enter by the back door and hugs the house's perimeter, like a soldier scouting enemy territory. I doubt she leaves the garden. But Willy gets bolder with every passing day. He quickly assumes control of the front, where he spends a lot of time lolling in the driveway, flirting with passersby, and perching on the porch rail to meow urgently—especially at 5:00 A.M., like an urban rooster—when he wants to be let in. Where he goes when he's outside is anybody's guess. Willy and Luna soon develop a warm-weather routine of staying out at night and dozing during the day inside or under the shade of a deck chair.

Of course, being pets, and not feral animals, their excursions are exclusively for fun. A study done at the University of Illinois Department of Natural Resources and Environmental Sciences by then-graduate student Jeff A. Horn confirms that outdoor pets wander a lot less than wild-living cats. Horn and his colleagues attached activity sensors to collars and then tracked the movements of forty-two cats, both owned and unowned, using radio telemetry. As might be expected, they found that pets usually stuck closer to home—generally within about two hectares—and that their movements betrayed a lack of urgency to their hunting. The feral kitties, on the other hand, roamed widely and were more aware of the environment, including potential dangers and the availability of prey. Unowned females had a home range of 60 hectares, and males almost 160 hectares.

Before collecting roaming data, Horn and his associates observed several cats for baseline activity levels. Predictably, they found that cats are world-class nappers. They spend about three-quarters of their time sleeping or "denning"; 20 percent in leisurely activities such as walking, grooming, or eating; and just 5 percent in highly active behaviors such as playing, capturing prey, and running. Human-attached felines with free access to the outdoors spent far less time in strenuous movement than unowned cats—3 percent versus 14 percent of their days. (One can only imagine how drastically vigorous activity drops off for indoor cats.) But while mapping their ranges is informative, it's only a proxy for how much exercise a cat actually gets. That's because feline movement is as much in the vertical as the horizontal plane. Cats climb, perch, and survey. They stalk, hide, and freeze. They chase, jump, and pounce. The beautiful curve of a seated cat owes itself to the animal's powerful haunches and strong back, both adaptations that allow it to spring several feet into the air.

The aerial aspect of their movements is good news for indoor cat owners who, at least in theory, if they adapt their homes for their pets, can thus encourage them to be more active. One of them is Elinor Karlsson, director of vertebrate genomics at the Broad Institute of MIT and Harvard. I hear, via the grapevine, that she has practically given over her home to creating a stimulating environment for her three cats. This is borne out in the first moments of our Zoom tour, when a gigantic running wheel—probably the size of a truck tire—rumbles into action behind her grinning face. A rangy, white cat has leaped on and gives it a couple spins before ambling off again. "Lacey's definitely the most active one. She's the one where the other cats will be crashed out somewhere fast asleep, and she'll be like—and what are we doing now? Where's the next excitement gonna come from? . . . She just loves anything new and exciting. So she uses the cat wheel all the time."

Karlsson shows me around her home. "I'm a little notorious when it comes to this," she acknowledges. She turns her camera on a pair of large windows that look onto a snowy, fenced-in backyard. "Can you see it up there? Above the window? That's the exit to my outdoor cat run." To get to the run, the cats climb to a landing and then nudge open a flap in the wall. Once outside, they can slink all around the edges of Karlsson's apartment walls, contained in spaces that look like horizontally laid ducts made from wire mesh. I am impressed. And curious. Do they use it a lot? All the time. Do they go out in the winter? They do. Where do you get this kind of equipment? (I don't seem to recall it on the shelf of my local PetSmart.) "There's a place up in Canada where you order it and they'll do all the [parts] custom. You tell them what you want, and they make different shapes and pieces, and then they ship it to you." The final component to Karlsson's extensive cat habitat is wall-mounted platforms at different heights, scratching posts, and several mysterious freestanding structures.

Still, the presence of all the specialized equipment has only been partially successful. "Right now I've got three cats; a skinny one, a medium-size one, and a fat one. . . . Lacey's very high energy." Hopper, the medium-size one, named after the early computer scientist Grace Hopper, not so much, although he uses the wheel "when he gets excited." And Beagle, the chubbette, who, continuing the science theme, was named after the ship Darwin used to visit the Galápagos Islands, is downright lethargic. "I should get him using it a bit more," Karlsson frets. Worried about his weight—although she believes it to be as much the result of overeating as inactivity, she tries to coax him into exercising by hiding dry food in an Egg-Cersizer Treat Dispenser, so he must chase and swat it to reach the kibbles.

Karlsson, who is smart, funny, and imaginative, is the perfect person to talk with for this book, and we keep going off on long, delightful tangents. She tells me her friend and colleague is working on a new definition of domestication, which depends on where on a spectrum a species falls in terms of their relationship with human beings. "What Kathryn [Lord, an animal behavior scientist, especially canine] has proposed is that basically, cats are completely domesticated because they can't compete successfully against other species without humans being around. So the food source, these little rodents they tend to eat, is outside of our houses. If the humans weren't around, they'd be competing with the foxes, they'd be competing with the coyotes, they'd be competing with all these other animals. I mean, you go up to Vermont and you don't see wild cats living in the woods. But with humans here, creating this little pocket for them where these other animals don't really want to be, all of a sudden they've got free rein to eat on small things. So, the evolutionary perspective, which is not warm and fuzzy at all, is that they clearly don't care about us being here and are possibly exploiting us."

Then we wander onto the topic I wanted to explore when I set up the interview, indoor versus outdoor cats. Karlsson has no doubts that keeping cats inside is the right thing to do morally and environmentally, since it minimizes their harm to birds. She also admits to a certain amount of convenience—she doesn't have to be concerned about ticks or fleas, about injuries or diseases from encounters with wildlife, or car accidents. But when she looks at it from the cat's side of the equation, she has misgivings. "The thing that worries me about it is that . . . it feels like at some point in time, that pet-care professionals made this decision that it was safer for cats to be inside. . . . But they didn't put as much emphasis on what you need to do to have a cat live an indoor life, and be fulfilled in the way that a cat needs to be. Because my cats would have a blast if they got outside. Lacey managed to sneak out the other day for like, the first time ever—and I'm paranoid, 'cause I know she'll love it out there—she thought it was like the best thing since sliced bread. I mean, it's super exciting out there . . . I do know that I am depriving them of something by not letting them out there: I'm depriving them of that ability to exhibit natural behaviors that they would love to be using." Her thought process recapitulates the logic of the cat chapter of the 2014 book *The Ethics of Captivity*, edited by Wesleyan University philosophy professor Lori Gruen, which, after a close examination, concludes that the argument that we keep cats indoors for their own good doesn't hold water—it is for our own. As Karlsson pointed out, we gain convenience and avoidance of loss, but, the authors suggest, for some, even many, cats, it is cruel. At the end of our conversation, Karlsson laughed, waving her hand behind her. Suddenly the cats, who'd been milling about aimlessly, stiffened, their noses pressed intently against the window: a rabbit. "As soon as the rabbit moves out of sight up here," she says, "they will charge down the basement stairs to look out the window downstairs." Although I'm happy to know that this bunny will continue to hip hop unhurriedly through the snow, I feel sorry for the cats, watching forever-out-of-reach prey and never, not even for one exultant minute, being able to tune every one of their keen senses and perfectly calibrated muscles to the single thing they were designed to do.

∞

This being America, the move to keep cats indoors was fueled by the invention of a new product: kitty litter. Until the 1940s, household felines used the great outdoor potty for their needs. If weather or health kept them in, owners provided a box filled with sand, sawdust, or ashes. However, the particles clung to paws, which left messes everywhere. In the winter of 1947, Michigan resident and navy veteran Edward Lowe was asked by his neighbor if he would give her a bit of sand from his coal, ice, and sawdust company for her pet. Instead, he offered her some Fuller's Earth, an absorbent clay. She liked it so much she came back for more—and brought some cat-owning friends with her. Lowe was soon selling five-pound bags at local stores, a business that he eventually sold for hundreds of millions of dollars. (Of course, a twenty-first-century environmental lens reveals a big downside to Tidy Cat; the clays are strip-mined and the used litter adds over two million tons to landfills annually.) The ability to take care of kitty's excretory needs inside, the mid-century discovery of spaying and neutering techniques and their popularization, and the advent of commercial pet food—canned food was introduced in the 1930s; dry kibbles ascended when, during World War II, the military requisitioned tin supplies—combined to drive roving felines indoors.

As someone going against the grain, I've given a lot of thought to the indoor-outdoor cat debate. So one frigid day in late January 2021, I invited our neighbor Miriam for a walk so I could learn more about her two indoor cats. We head off toward the river, chitchatting about our children (her daughter has just returned to Ohio to live with friends and study remotely at Oberlin) and work (I am in the middle of an intense campaign for the COVID-19 vaccine-hesitant). We cross the parkway at a crosswalk and then head left. Lone runners and pairs of bundled-up walkers pass us going the other direction. I already went running, which I've noticed leaves me warm for the entire day, but the additional activity raises my temperature even more, and I'm soon perspiring in my light coat and sweater. At the bridge, we consider—return or keep going along the highway? We keep going, and I get ready to broach the topic of her decision to keep their cats indoors. Miriam is thoughtful and sensitive—I always enjoy our conversations, so I expect her to delve into their reasoning with relish. Instead, she becomes visibly distressed and tells me it's something they never thought about. I assure her that I plan to write a well-balanced chapter—outlining the real risks and benefits to both sides. The dangers for outdoor cats are well-known, I say, but there are disadvantages for indoor cats, too, starting with lifestyle diseases and ending with behavior issues related to boredom, frustration, and the stress of being in close quarters with other cats. But it is clear she feels judged.

Nothing could be further from the case. Miriam is one of the most conscientious people I know. She is my preferred cat-sitter when we go away for the weekend. Despite our glaring philosophical differences regarding *Felis catus*, she and Greg fell in love with our new kittens, especially Willy, who they saluted when they passed our house, sometimes pausing to sit on our railroad ties with him purring on their laps. (Fascinatingly, this soothing sound, a hallmark of domestication—and known to help human healing—can only be made by sacrificing the ability to roar. Purrers have fused hyoid bones in the throats. Roarers have flexible ones so they can open their jaws wide to scare the bejesus out of us.) With Miriam at the helm, I turn the key and don't look back, knowing that my extraordinarily competent friend will manage every detail. She will cope with our always malfunctioning alarm—sometimes the number of bypasses to enter is so long, it feels like an old-fashioned adding machine. Her empathy leads her to arrive on the dot for Willy and Luna's feedings since she worries about them going hungry, and diligently scoop their poop from the litter box I've left in the downstairs bathroom, because she sympathizes with their revulsion at dirtying themselves.

As we stride along in the foggy, darkening afternoon, she describes her daily routine with her own cats, which only underscores her high level of consideration for any sentient being. Both were rescues: Loki, gray and fluffy, and Parvati, a pure black shorthair that experienced early trauma and remains skittish. They have free range of Miriam's two-story house and even their own "bathroom," a closet where any leavings are whisked away within hours. Each cat has her own special diet, tailored to her individual nutritional needs by a veterinarian. They have many toys and are given regular workouts with a teaser, a stick with a feather or small object tied to it with a string. Yet, over the years, the girls have put on extra weight, and Loki has developed diabetes, requiring daily insulin injections. Miriam and I come to another turning point and decide to further extend our walk—in the end we've tramped four and a half miles. The cat's illness has become the organizing principle of her life—she schedules her meetings so she can be home to administer the injections and hires a house sitter when she travels.

Indoor cat owners want what's best for their kitties. But at the same time, there are definite health impacts of permanent confinement—not the least of which is obesity. To find out more about how professionals view the trade-offs, I arranged to talk to one of the owners of a clinic where I have occasionally brought our cats. Frank Trudeau always wanted to be a veterinarian. But then in college he watched a neuter surgery and got queasy—for four years. Eventually, he recovered enough to take some classes in organic chemistry and biochemistry and enrolled in the Tufts School of Veterinary Medicine. Since then, he's worked at Best Friends Animal Hospital in Melrose, Massachusetts, a local practice with a waiting room so cramped that clients' knees practically touch on the L-shaped bench. Like most small-animal practices, Best Friends sees a steady stream of dogs and cats, spiced by the occasional bunny, bird, or guinea pig. Trudeau, an affable man in his forties, especially likes the fact that every day is different. In part, this is because their clientele, drawn from the surrounding area, is solidly working and middle class, and tend to be devoted, but not rolling-in-it, pet owners. They often opt for in-house treatment rather than go to expensive specialists. But, Trudeau notes with a grimace, veterinary work "can be very stressful. It's one of those careers with high rates of compassion fatigue and suicide." I'm momentarily taken aback. But, of course. "Every week we euthanize several animals. . . . A lot of vets, they own their clinic, they're running a business, they're trying to see animals, they're trying to manage people. And that can be stressful."

Trudeau walks me through an average day, which, unexpectedly, involves a lot of dental work. "Yeah, so the spays and neuters are pretty routine, but we never know how long it's gonna take once we start doing teeth. That sometimes is a very quick procedure. And sometimes it's like, hours, hours, and hours of grunt work. Because we just don't know how bad it's going to be. It's probably the number one disease we see." He then lists all the ills that can befall a pet's oral hygiene: tartar, gum inflammation, gingivitis, and periodontal disease. I wince guiltily when he bemoans that many people resist tooth-brushing, recalling my decision to decline the $13 tube of salmon-flavored toothpaste and diminutive toothbrush recommended for one of our cats.

"Do you think it has something to do with their diets?" I ask him. "In earlier times, a dog or cat's diet had bones and cartilage and stuff that might have scoured their teeth clean?" Trudeau isn't convinced. His theory is that as dog breeding has sought miniatures and striking facial features, canine jaws have become too small for the mouthful of choppers they inherited from their ancestors. "Now if you have a little dog, you have all these teeth that are rotated and crowded, they were bred to have a smushed-in skull." But, he allows, the carb-heavy commercial pet food might have something to do with it.

Like most veterinary medicine practitioners and researchers, Trudeau blames poor quality food and too much of it for the pet obesity epidemic that has paralleled the human one. He says that about half the dogs and cats they see in their practice are overweight and almost a third are outright obese. Every month, he says, they diagnose new cases of diabetes and other lifestyle diseases. This jibes with national and international statistics. A 2018 survey by the Association for Pet Obesity Prevention (APOP) found that 60 percent of cats were overweight and obese. This makes them prone to diabetes; a British survey of almost two hundred thousand cats found that one in two hundred had the disease. Fat cats also have higher rates of hyperthyroidism—1.5–11.4 percent of older cats, according to the *Journal of Feline Medicine and Surgery*—and dental disease. Dog statistics show them to be similarly corpulent. The APOP survey puts the rate at 56 percent, and in 2019, over half of the canines seen at the one thousand Banfield Pet Hospitals, the nation's largest veterinary clinic chain, were overweight or obese. Like curvy kitties, heavy hounds are prone to diabetes, heart disease, hypertension, and degenerative joint diseases.

Just like with people, veterinarians take a diet-centered approach to solving the pet adiposity crisis. Laments Trudeau, "Dry food just isn't the right thing for cats. . . . So that's one thing we do with a diabetic or obese cat is we get them off dry food and get them on the higher protein, lower-carb food. And with dogs, always the problem is, you know, the grand-parent or the kids spoiling the dog, throwing food on the floor. Or just, you know, too much quantity on the kibbles." Also just like with people, animal health professionals focus on bickering about optimal weight loss plans. "Experts . . . disagree on which type of food promotes better weight loss, wet or dry," explains a 2018 article in the *New York Times* about fat dogs and cats. "Some data suggests wet food's higher water and protein content carries more benefit because it reduces appetite," says the scientist they cite, veterinary nutritionist Jonathan Stockman. "But dry food has a higher fiber content, he says, so a similar argument can be made for that. 'One really is no better than the other,' Dr. Stockman says. 'We usually go with prescription diets because the nutrient density can be controlled and you can cut calories without causing a nutritional deficiency.'" (As usual, the only winner here is the pet food industry. APOP claims on its Facebook page to receive no industry funding, but in 2014 Purina Cat Chow said it would donate $50,000 to the organization if one hundred thousand cat owners signed the "Why Weight?" pledge.)

"Okay," I ask Trudeau. "So how about the other side of the equation. What percentage of your patients do you think get enough exercise and what percentage don't?" He doesn't know. Why? Because, just as with most human medical examinations, there is no way to assess physical fitness and no routine questions to document activity habits. (The standard measure of obesity for a small animal is to eyeball its physique and run your hands along its sides. If it has a tucked waist and not too much padding around the ribs, the cat or dog is considered to be at a healthy weight.) Still, Trudeau does his best to answer my question. "That's very hard to say. Owners with the big dogs are generally really active with the dog, but not so much with the smaller lap dogs. We don't go into super detail on that. I mean, if they're overweight, we ask. But if the dog looks reasonably lean, we don't go into too much detail on that. So, I'm not sure."

Because of the potential health benefits to humans, scientists have collected some data on dog walking. A 2014 review of thirty-one of these studies found that canines got 160 minutes a week of exercise during an average of four excursions. The authors note, "The exercise levels of dogs correlates well with their owners' activity levels and the exercise levels of dogs has been shown to be inversely associated with dog obesity, an increasing animal welfare issue." They go on to observe, however, that "a large proportion of the community who own a dog do not walk it or do so only occasionally. . . . It is estimated that only sixty percent of dog owners walk their dog at all." As with cats, a lack of physical activity can lead to canine behavior problems, including barking, destroying things around the house, aggression, pulling on the leash, disobedience, fear of strangers and loud noises, and escaping. Although I could find no scientific research on how to measure dog fitness, cardiovascular or muscular, or a recommended minimum daily level of moderate or vigorous activity for canine health, sources as diverse as the military, kennel clubs, and the makers of FitBark, the doggie equivalent of FitBit, concur that most breeds need at least one half hour walk daily, and some—retrievers, collies, and German shepherds, the types most often used for working or herding—need a good, solid hour or two of running, jumping, and other intense exertion.

Trudeau paints an equally bleak picture on the feline front. "With cats, well, we don't have many outdoor ones in this area, near the city. And you can't exercise them. You can play with them for a minute. But they'll stop when they're bored. So cats are kind of in charge of that. Sometimes we'll have people do the puzzle feeder. . . . Otherwise, laser pointers and all that stuff for exercise, but it's very hard." There is no national US data on animal physical activity, but a 2011 survey done by the Canadian Veterinary Medical Association in partnership with Hill's Pet Nutrition found that "veterinarians believe that the majority of dogs (55%) and cats (70%) they see do not receive an adequate amount of exercise to maintain good health."

"Do you think that being an indoor cat may be a contributor to the feline obesity and diabetes that you see?" I ask.

"Yes, I'm sure it is. Indoor cats are heavier. Outdoor cats, or cats that are only kept indoors in the winter, are leaner, especially in the summer when they're going out." As if uneasy even suggesting that cats might do better with regular access to nature, Trudeau hastens to remind me of the many dangers they face outside. He doesn't have to. The unequivocal recommendation of the Veterinary Medicine Association of America is for cats to be kept inside. "Free-roaming cats may have a reduced life span and be exposed to injury, suffering, and death from vehicles; attacks from other animals; euthanasia; human cruelty; poisons; traps; and weather extremes," the organization's website states. This norm has created a rancorous divide among cat owners. Our family, squarely in the outdoor camp, is in the much-vilified minority. Once, when Luna was young and hadn't returned within a couple hours, I posted to Nextdoor asking if anyone had seen her. This detonated a heated debate, none of which centered on finding her. Luckily, she soon showed up and, after giving Willy the customary front and backend sniff, insouciantly sauntered to the food bowl. Some indoor-cat advocates are in the habit of treating any cat they encounter, especially ones without collars—as most of ours end up being (what else is a breakaway collar good for?)—as a stray, reporting them to animal control or, as happened during some of the three saddest days of Esme's early childhood, kidnapping them. (We reclaimed our feline with an ever-widening dragnet of posters, at last finding her four blocks away at the house of a woman who claimed to have "mistaken" her for one of her own dozen and a half indoor cats.) But like Miriam's clowder, most of our neighbors' cats never leave their homes.

❧

Willy and Luna were rebound relationships. The September before we got them, our twelve-year-old cat Smokey had died of lung cancer, the most devastating loss of Mariela's life. Originally, Smokey had been a consolation prize for Esme. After seven blissful years of being an only child, over the course of eighteen months, she'd acquired two younger sisters. Rafi and I, too overwhelmed by constant infant and toddler care to even be able to sit down with her, watched her world implode from afar. No longer the object of extravagant cuddles; long, rambling conversations; and late-night storytelling sessions, our shell-shocked oldest daughter withdrew. We did the only thing we could think of to cheer her up: We got her a kitten. As if imitating Rafi's and my absorption with her siblings, Smokey became a permanent fixture in Esme's arms, tucked into the crook of an elbow with her soft, gray belly exposed. They were so conjoined that even the fact that I filled the food dish did nothing to win more than an icy stare.

For years, Smokey regarded the rest of us with suspicion, if not outright hostility. She kept her distance and channeled her disdain into shredding our furniture. (I have privately bestowed on her the title of Most Destructive Cat Ever. I estimate, between ripped lace curtains, torn velvet upholstery, and ragged office chairs, some $10,000 in damages.) But after Esme left for college, Smokey no longer had a protector. Enter Mariela, aka the cat whisperer. She poured herself into the task, which required countless bags of cat treats, innumerable repetitions of simple commands such as "sit" and "lie," and, after all else had failed, "help" in the form of a firm shove. Smokey resolutely resisted training, but she flourished in the attention. Within a couple months, she'd transferred her attachment to Mariela and become more accepting of the rest of us. Soon, even my mother, who, although she loves cats, had never warmed to Smokey (might have had something to do with those curtains), began to refer to the two of them as "the old ladies of the house." She enjoyed commenting that Smokey seemed as stiff and arthritic as she was, but lately had started to toll a warning. "I don't think Smokey's doing well. I may outlast her after all."

I could be biased, but there is no more Edenic spot than our backyard. What is most incredible about it is that it all came out of Rafi's brain. After the contractor we'd hired to build a wheelchair-accessible, ground-floor bedroom and bathroom battered down with his massive-wheeled excavator all but a few trees, flattened our flowerbeds, and extended the footprint of the house twenty feet further into our already runty lot, the girls and I cried. What was left of their small but green childhood retreat was a deep pit, mounds of dirt, some broken concrete, and a few stumps. "Don't worry, it's going to be better than ever," Rafi said. No one was reassured. He plunged into the project the way he does every-thing: headfirst, all systems go, and no safety net. For weeks, he nattered on about perc rates, gradients, dry wells, and French drains, boring me and irritating the contractor—especially when he insisted that he lay a vapor barrier before he poured the concrete floor to protect it against the—surprise! surprise!—water table in which it was sitting. He made numerous trips to Home Depot and New England Gravel, returning with the minivan sagging with peastone or brimming with PVC pipes, a modern-day mule laden with firewood. He explained that his drainage system would keep our house, with its 150-year-old fieldstone foundation, airtight. He then proceeded to tote in truckfuls of soil, cobblestones, bricks, and railroad ties, and with the help of a cast of rotating characters from the local day-labor pool (my job was to provide a hearty almuerzo, the standard perk of intra–Latin American employment), graded a terraced garden crossed by sloping brick walkways and filled with inviting patios and shady nooks. He even left an area in a newly sunny corner for a lawn.

The garden is the perfect spot for celebrations, like the birthday party we had for Esmerelda when she turned twenty-one. She had just started classes after spending her second semester of junior year in a study-abroad program in Sevilla, Spain, and the summer as an intern for a World Health Organization tuberculosis program in Geneva, Switzerland. But she came by for a couple hours, and we all sat around our slatted eucalyptus table. My mother, dressed in a lilac linen shift and pink stone beads, at the head, radiating contentment through a glass of white wine; Rafi, the two younger girls, and I along the sides; and Esme opposite her grandmother, regaling us with anecdotes about her travels and inviting us to help her brainstorm for her senior thesis. Smokey lay nearby in the grass, a dim spot in the green. The sun trickled through the tree branches and we dawdled over our meal, cake, and presents. Here we all are, together, I thought. For how long?

Even that afternoon, as we took our places under the heart-shaped redbud leaves and clusters of red crab apples, Smokey had arrived last. When she got there, she lowered herself painfully to the ground. Her topaz eyes skimmed our faces, but her breathing rasped and caught. A couple weeks earlier, we'd brought her to the vet. She had gotten very thin; her coat was dull and straggly; and her cute snore, Mariela's nightly lullaby, had become closer to a chainsaw buzz. We saw Dr. O'Grady, a former circus vet who now worked at Best Friends Animal Hospital. He listened to us describe her symptoms, examined her, and took some X-rays. Smokey had lung cancer, he told us, and was quite far along. We could treat, but it would be difficult for her and would probably not prolong her life. The best option might be palliative. As we sang "Happy Birthday," and Esme blew out the candles, I watched the cat's thin ribs stutter. The time had come. Instead of suffering in her final moments, we would help her leave the world painlessly. After the meal, I sent out frantic emails. (Why do emergencies always happen on holidays?) I arranged for euthanasia the following day at a twenty-four-hour veterinary hospital. Now to tell the kids.

I expected Esme and Mariela to be devastated, but not Gabi, who was never an animal lover. She hates dogs, an antipathy born as a boisterous toddler when her continual running led her to be singled out as the object of several high-speed canine chases (one involving pit bulls). At four, she'd been traumatized by our stay at a relative's hacienda in Ecuador, where the servants hissingly warned her that if she didn't finish her food, she would be fed to Mateo, a devilish-looking black bulldog with red-rimmed eyes. She kept Smokey at arm's length, neither addressing nor patting her, and was singularly uninterested in touching the sheep, ponies, and cows at our favorite petting zoo. But when I delivered the news that we had an appointment to put Smokey to sleep, she burst into tears. For the next three hours, my middle child, who is usually as reserved as her sisters are open, poured out her innermost thoughts. Smokey had been there for as long as Gabi could remember. She was part of the family. She couldn't die. What would that mean about her childhood? About the home—crazy and tumultuous, but familiar and constant—she assumed would always be there? What would it mean about us? I have never seen her so anguished, not even when, five years earlier, she had witnessed her grandfather die in agony of pancreatic cancer.

The ancient Egyptians, who revered cats, would have understood the intensity of her feelings. Although only the pharaoh could officially own a cat, families that shared their homes with felines grieved the deaths of their pets as deeply as they did those of humans. They shaved their eyebrows to show they were in mourning. They dressed the undersized corpses with oils and scents, and wrapped them in linen patterned to suggest their striped coats and with "painted faces depicting quizzical, almost humorous, expressions," according to religion scholar Alleyn Diesel. They even buried them with people, or in special cat graveyards, in which archeologists say "the soil in some places is almost solid dried cat," reports geographer James Allen Baldwin. Cats abound in ancient Egyptian art. They are depicted confronting rodents, accompanying humans on bird-hunting trips, crouched under chairs, or tending to their young. The goddess Bastet, often portrayed as a slender woman with a cat head, was the guardian of the home, of women, and of pregnancy and childbirth. Scientists believe the Egyptians shaped modern cats' personalities. "They would have selected for the ones that were easiest to have around—more social and less territorial than their predecessors," says Carlos Driscoll of the World Wildlife Fund in a 2017 article in *Science*.

The cats who share our homes may have been domesticated multiple times; feline remains have been found in human settlements in Cypress, in a dig dating to 8000 B.C.E. and in ancient Egypt, around 3000 B.C.E. Their ancestors were small wild cats, *Felis libyca*, who, the theory goes, were attracted by the vermin that plagued crops and food stores once people started farming. Humans, appreciative that the consummate hunters kept rodent populations down, may have encouraged them by leaving them food. Eventually, as the two species got more comfortable with each other, the cats braved the indoors. As Karlsson's friend had noted in her theory on the spectrum of domestication, this gave cats a huge evolutionary advantage: not only did living with people provide a steady source of prey, supplemented by the occasional tidbit, but their houses and outbuildings offered a protected environment for cats to bear and rear their young. (The proof is in the pudding: there are now an estimated four hundred million cats worldwide.) Of course, when it comes to living with humans, cats have nothing on dogs, who have been panting at our sides for the past fifteen to thirty thousand years, easily winning first place for earliest domesticated animal. Dogs are known to be extremely sensitive to human emotions, and both pet and owner gush oxytocin, the "love hormone," when gazing into each other's eyes. The two species remain popular today; some two-thirds of Americans have a pet.

These animals are fixtures in our households, the patient objects of myriad caresses, in service to our need to be soothed, calmed, and cuddled. (I've proposed the term *love slaves* to my family and friends, but so far the response has been tepid.) In the spellbinding 1978 documentary *Gates of Heaven*, an unlikely film about the pet cemetery business, the owner of Bubbling Well Pet Memorial Park observes that pets fulfill our "need to have something to fondle," and that they are essentially replacement children. He postulates that the explosion in animal caring was driven by working couples who postpone childbearing and lonely grandparents who no longer live in multigenerational settings. (The facts, at least more recent ones, do not bear this out; a 2003 Humane Society study found that the life stage most likely to have a pet was "middle parents," at almost three-quarters of all households, although they are closely followed by young couples, at 72.5 percent.)

Cats and dogs are both members of a carnivorous branch of the tree of life; however, in their long association with humans, dogs evolved to eat a diet similar to ours. Unlike their wild cousins, such as wolves and coyotes, dogs easily digest and metabolize starches, such as wheat and rice, setting them up right for tableside scrap scrounging. "Dogs are different from wolves and don't need a wolflike diet," comments dog evolutionary biologist Robert Wayne in an article in *Science*. "They have coevolved with humans and their diet." This difference came to a head a few years ago when, following the human low-carb trend, pet owners began feeding their canine friends expensive grain-free kibbles with names like Arcana, Zignature, and Taste of the Wild. Suddenly, hundreds of dogs died of canine dilated cardiomyopathy (DCM), a rare heart condition. In July 2018, the FDA began investigating the reports, concluding that there was some dietary link, although it required more research to know exactly what it was.

Cats, who earned their hearthside spot by keeping rodent populations in check, need no such alimentary supplementation. They remain hypercarnivores—requiring a diet that is more than 70 percent protein and fat; to support this, their digestive system consists of a relatively larger stomach and smaller bowel, since most of their digestion is chemical, or enzyme-based. There, they break down protein and fat, but have very few enzymes for digesting carbohydrates, either in their mouths or intestines. And since sugar does little for them nutritionally, they do not taste sweetness. "Despite the poor capacity of the domestic cat to utilize diets with significant levels of carbohydrate, many commercial cat diets contain relatively high levels of carbohydrate. For cats maintained on these diets, it is likely that rodents, small birds, etc. are an absolute dietary requirement," write William H. Karasov, a forest and wildlife ecologist, and Angela E. Douglas, an entomologist, in *Comparative Digestive Physiology*.

This makes me feel somewhat better about the enthusiastic hunters we've sheltered over the years, all of whom have made regular offerings to the family food basket in the form of freshly slaughtered field mice on the doormat or, as was Smokey's specialty, brought in alive and released for some romping indoor fun. While I confess to a certain indifference to rodent death, I feel differently about the very occasional songbird—always a fledgling who's failed its maiden flight, which is why I don't hang birdfeeders in the warm months. (I've never seen a cat catch a squirrel—probably something to do with their acrobatic ability to balance on narrow branches and even telephone lines.) Yet it seems delusional—even harmful—to deny a feline its nature. Like us, cats are contradictory. Dainty mouths and noses and immense, limpid eyes are harnessed to sharp teeth and retractable claws. A yearning for affection and a firm attachment to the group—our cats trail us from room to room and join all our social gatherings—are paired with annihilating blood thirst. We may bliss out in long sessions of cuddling, stroking, gazing, and vocalizations (them, purrs; us, baby talk). Later that same day, they may chase a baby bunny down the basement stairs, trapping it at the bottom, and then slowly dismember it, leaving the yard gruesomely decorated with bits of hide, intestines and organs, and a fragment of face. To truly love a cat is to accept the duality of their natures—and thus our own.

∽

After Smokey died, our house felt dark and all the activity in it perfunctory. The girls went to school. Rafi and I worked in our basement offices. My mother, whose mobility and ability to care for herself were gravely impaired at that point, mostly stayed in her large tree-shaded addition, visited by an infinite procession of nurses, aides, and physical, occupational, and speech therapists. At midday, I would hear her drag herself into the kitchen—one leg barely worked, so it was step, scrape, step, scrape, like a badly injured frog—braced on her walker, to get some yogurt or fruit from the one shelf in the refrigerator she could reach now that she was so stooped and frail. But I didn't hear her voice, muffled and scratchy from Parkinson's, talking to Smokey as she wove around her walker, curled snoozing on a chair, or meowed at the door. Far worse, Mariela, whose joyful nature is as irrepressible as a carbon dioxide bubble, was deflated. As the youngest, both in a large family and in a small gang of neighborhood girls, she'd never needed to make outside friends—why should she when she was already part of two clamorous groups? But now her sister and neighborhood friends, the people with whom she'd spent every afternoon and weekend, were high school students. They did dance, theater, sports, and clubs, activities that kept them busy until dinner. Mariela had always been content alone—she was prone to creative bursts where she'd suddenly hand-sew dozens of stuffed animals or fold and decorate armies of paper boxes. But now there was no one her age around and her most faithful companion was gone. Her smile got pinched, and her chatter dwindled. A couple nights a week, the bedroom door would swing open and Mariela would climb into our king-size bed, startling us awake. "I miss Smokey's snores." "Best cat ever," I would say, and then we'd cry, the grief clogging our throats and prickling our eyes.

We mourned for months until, in early winter, Mariela told us she was finally ready for another cat. We tested the waters by fostering an adult rescue. He was a bulky brown-and-white tom, who had obviously been maltreated—he'd been found living near a restaurant dumpster, and the rescue organization wondered if he might have been tortured. He was starved for attention, so he clung to our heels. But he was so jumpy that unless we moved as if we were doing tai chi, he would cuff our legs with his long, sharp nails. Only my mother, who inched along with her walker, was slow enough to be reassuring. We tried to accommodate his needs, but one night he viciously attacked Mariela's shins as she rearranged them on her bed, raking his claws across her skin, leaving deep incisions and drawing a lot of blood. Against her pleading, I decided he would have to go. Our next attempt, we decided, would have to be a kitten. Mariela began to trawl the cat adoption pages like someone with an online shopping addiction and soon found two kittens that a nearby facility required be adopted together, since they had, in the clinical way we describe nonhuman love, "bonded" in their foster home. Although I'd planned to get just one, after seeing pictures of the two intertwined, their light and dark coats like a living yin and yang, I quickly acquiesced. It felt like unexpected bounty from the universe to welcome them both into our home.

The first few days, as advised by the rescue organization, we kept them enclosed in a small space while they got their bearings. In our case, my mother's new wheelchair-accessible bathroom on the main floor. As soon as we lifted the grate to their carrier, Willy strutted out to explore the tiled space from top to bottom. Luna, however, had to be pulled out—and then ran and hid behind the plastic shower curtain. Mariela sat on the floor and waited. Eventually, after he'd investigated his surroundings, Willy marched onto her lap. Luna stood back, but after a while, she climbed on, too. Mariela stroked them gently, inhaling the fragile, warm scent of kitten. In no time flat, they became a threesome, dozing in a pile, grooming any furry (or hairless) body part in range, and greeting each other effusively. My youngest was happier than I'd seen her in a long time.

For a month, life was perfect. Everyone was doing well. It was May, which, with its warmth, profusion of new leaves, and fragrant flowers—verbena, lilacs, lilies of the valley, and roses—has always seemed to embody hope. And we were looking forward to two major events that would happen over a single weekend: Esmerelda's graduation from college, attended by her immediate family, and my mother's eightieth birthday, for which all her children and grandchildren would convene briefly at our house before going to my mother's girlhood home in Vermont, so four sets of her early friends could attend. Esme's graduation was dampened slightly by pouring rain, but afterward the five of us went to a Mexican restaurant. Rafi brought my mother separately in our sedan, since it's the only vehicle low enough for her to get into without being carried. On the way, Rafi, who never censors what crosses his mind, wondered if she was ready to die. "Yes," she told him. She did that weekend, on the morning of the day that was to be her birthday party.

∽

Luna is perplexed. She sniffs the imitation leather lounge chair in Rafi's basement office, hunching her slight spine. Then she scurries to the door, waiting to be let out. A few minutes later, she scratches to be let in. She returns to the chair, inhales sharply several times. The chair is one of Willy's many napping spots. Where is he?

After my mother died, the patter of their tiny feet masked the quiet where she had once been, slowly rasping across the floor or calling us to help her. We lifted them to our faces and felt the thrum of their small hearts. Although our family had been slashed—a week after her grandmother's death, Esmerelda had moved to California for her first post-college job, Willy and Luna brightened the house—and our spirits. We were grateful for their calligraphic forms, their dignified affection shown by winding through our ankles or purring, and our easy and respectful coexistence. Rafi developed an extra special relationship with Willy, carrying him about like a toddler, his legs hanging loosely down, and addressing him as Willy My Boy. The son he never once said he wished we'd had? Or an increased appreciation for life's fragility after facing the deaths of three parents in five years?

Willy had become the king of the block. Outside, he sat imperiously in front of our house where he could survey the road and solicit attention. I'd often glance out the window, as I washed dishes or watered plants, and see a stranger stooping to pat him. He ranged down the street, making early morning visits to our neighbors. He also seemed to get more and more comfortable with cars, sitting placidly on the railroad ties while our minivan entered the driveway and crossing the street to mosey along the abutting side street. "Willy, shoo," I scolded him. "You're a backyard cat." But only Luna truly was. She refused to set foot on the sidewalk and rarely attempted the front porch.

"Why is Luna acting so strange?" I asked Rafi.

"Willy didn't come for breakfast." Over the summer, he'd shifted from his self-appointed 5:30 A.M. wake-up duties to a just-in-time arrival at 7:00 A.M. when Rafi went downstairs to brew coffee. It was as if he were having wonderful adventures from which it was difficult to pull away—even for one of his favorite activities, eating. Then I remembered I hadn't seen him the night before. We quickly realized he'd gone missing. I checked his usual haunts—beds, furniture, the clothes heaped on the floor of the laundry closet. No Willy. Rafi began to stroll the neighborhood, while I called Animal Control. No, they didn't have any yellow shorthairs. I rapidly posted a note and photos that he was missing on Nextdoor and a neighborhood Google group. Within twenty minutes a woman called. She was so very sorry. She'd seen a cat that looked like Willy hit during morning traffic the previous day on a street nearby. "No," I moaned, sinking to the floor. I called Animal Control back. "Have you had any reports of cats being hit by cars?"

"Let me look at the Department of Public Works log. Hold on a sec. Yes, there was a yellow striped tabby picked up yesterday." Rafi and I collapsed into each other's arms.

With our pet's death, I saw Rafi cry more than with either of his parents'. Human love is always complicated by the endless stories we tell to understand ourselves—nervous chatter that distracts more than it explains. But the love between species is mute and cannot be deflected. We can only watch each other, sit by each other, stroke fur, or lick a hand. We are silent witnesses to their brief time on this planet, and they to ours.

∽

In winter, Luna has the habit of standing at the back door and then, once she's sniffed the frosty air, retreating into the warm dining room.

A minute later, she's at the door again, a behavior that I concede may reveal some significant deficits when it comes to learning and reasoning. It also illustrates, we discover amid much laughter over dinner one night, basic differences in our characters: Rafi and Gabi impatiently nudge her out with a toe; Mariela and I wait, cold wind wafting in, as she makes up her mind. But never once, even after we'd realized Willy had been run over, have we denied her access to the outdoors. This is not always an easy choice; when she occasionally doesn't come when called or is late to a meal, I plummet into a worry spiral, sprinting around the house to make sure she isn't locked into a bedroom and repeatedly rattling the large plastic kibble container in the yard and on the walkways. But—forgive me, all my indoor-cat-owning friends—the alternative is not a life. Even if her thread is cut short by a speeding car or, our most recent addition to the local, urban wildlife, a marauding coyote, Luna is a happy cat. She picks her way through the snow or snoozes under a blueberry bush. She chases mayflies, sharpens her nails on the dogwood, prowls on a warm spring night. She eats when she's hungry, naps when she's tired, and cuddles with anyone who will have her (especially when, as with Rafi, there's a cozy beard involved). As we are all born to be, she is autonomous, in motion, and connected to nature.

Although I accept the heartbreaking risks of having an outdoor cat in the city as inevitable, Karlsson reminds me that this is a problem of our own making. "I bike everywhere. So I should point out—I don't particularly like cars. The thing that fascinates me about our lives, our children's lives, and our pets' lives is how much of them are shaped by the fact that we have allowed cars to completely dominate. Like the dogs-having-to-be-on-leashes-all-the-time thing—you can't take the risk of a dog moving away from you or running into the street. Or a child. We're all so constrained by that." Of course! Belatedly, our city lowered the speed limit to twenty miles per hour on the road where Willy was killed; at that pace, anyone can brake for an errant cat—or a bunny, wild turkey, child, or elder. What would it be like if our built environments weren't centered around the automobile? I fantasize about a future in which a combination of increased public spaces, more dedicated lanes for bicycles and pedestrians, and additional traffic-calming measures allow people—and their pets—to move freely.

3

The Fault Isn't in Our Food

M y tenth year was not a happy one. My family had just moved from a married student housing complex—my father went to graduate school at the ancient age of thirty—where the gated road teemed with playmates and games. The kids were a ragtag, international bunch, hailing from Mexico, Thailand, Israel, and Nigeria, as well as all over the United States. No one cared how old you were or whether you were a girl or a boy. The only important thing was to be able to run fast and for hours, as we spontaneously formed teams for tag, cops and robbers, hide-and-go-seek, kickball, whiffle ball, and street hockey.

But in the new neighborhood, there was no one my age, and while we had a house with a small fenced-in yard, the busy street was off-limits for sports. That year, my life narrowed to a dull but debilitating routine: After walking to and from the school about a half a mile away, I settled into an armchair, plowing through piles of library books and a family-sized bag of Nacho Doritos. By midyear, I'd accumulated twenty-five extra pounds. Even my new fashion statement—roomy engineer's overalls worn with a jaunty, red kerchief—couldn't hide the fact that I'd propelled myself firmly across the line from stocky to chubby.

For decades afterward, I blamed my weight gain on the chips. With over thirty ingredients, most of which were flavorings and dyes, almost half of total calories from fat, and diabolically engineered to override satiety, they seemed the most likely villain. Today, most experts and the public agree: energy-dense junk foods are a modern-day scourge, supplanting traditional healthful foods with mindless and endless snacking that has layered us with lard. But true to my contrarian nature, I've begun to rethink my apocryphal Doritos-made-me-fat story. The truth, I suspected, had little to do with the actual foodstuff—I could have been pounding sticks of butter, the treat I helped myself to on baby's first trip to the grocery store—and more to do with the fact that I'd replaced hours of physical activity with hours of immobility and, relatedly, was consuming more calories than I burned. With this in mind, I began to revisit our sanctimonious horror at processed food in general and "junk food," with its minimal nutritional contribution, in particular.

"Since 1960, the prevalence of adult obesity in the United States has nearly tripled, from thirteen percent in 1960–1962 to 36 percent during 2009–2010," states a Centers for Disease Control (CDC) study. From that point, the obesity rate has continued to climb, reaching 42.4 percent of the adult population in 2017–2018. Could this well-documented worldwide widening of the waistline be my story writ large (groan)? Let's take a closer look at industrial food from a health perspective, to see if there's any evidence that it has special obesity and disease-imparting qualities, or if the problem is as simple as it's always been thought to be: eating too much and moving too little.

Opponents claim processed food is brimming with deleterious substances. These come in two general categories. First, some specific ingredients, such as sugar and high fructose corn syrup (HFCS) or fat, saturated fat, and trans fat, are said to have unique properties making them harmful over and above their caloric contribution. Second, practically any additive that has a polysyllabic name is viewed with suspicion and fear by the public, food activists, and many researchers—in fact, pretty much anyone who isn't a food scientist or technologist! Happily, most of these assertions have proved to be untrue.

Although there have been exhaustive studies, scientists have mostly been unable to document a special obesity-inducing quality, nor, with one exception, an incontrovertible disease link, in specific foodstuffs. (The one exception is trans fat, the unnaturally shaped molecules of which stud arterial walls and contribute to plaque formation.)

For years, fat, and especially saturated fat, was the villain du jour. A post–World War II spike in heart disease was attributed to the good life enjoyed by the white-collar professionals who shuttled between their urban offices and suburban homes in zaftig automobiles; wooed clients with three-martini, steak, and *pomme frites* lunches; and on weekends participated in endless rounds of competitive cocktailing and grilling. The bottom began to fall out of that theory at the turn of the twenty-first century, when researchers, whose biochemical identification tools now allowed them to differentiate among a whole range of blood molecules, found that intake of saturated fats, while it might increase total cholesterol, didn't necessarily correspond to increases in the least healthy types of molecules (low-density lipoprotein, LDL). Health authorities, while they haven't advocated a wholehearted return to smearing pats of butter on everything, now suggest people include ample healthy fats, such as those from plants and fish, in their diets.

More recently, blame has turned to sugar. There are two accusations. First, that fructose, which is metabolized by the liver, also damages it and increases blood cholesterol and insulin resistance. Fructose is used widely in soda and as a sweetener for bakery products and condiments. Says George Bray, one of the founders of the field of obesity studies, "Nonalcoholic fatty liver disease did not exist when I was a medical student. It appeared in the 1980s, and it is now a significant precursor, if not the leading one, of end-stage liver disease and liver transplants. The consumption of soft drinks had doubled by the 1980s. This suggests to me that the rising intake of fructose in soft drinks could play a role in the development of nonalcoholic fatty liver disease." The other allegation is that sugar, because it is so calorically dense and easy to consume—think the aforementioned soda and fruit juices, contributes disproportionately to obesity.

The United States, unlike the European Union and the international community, doesn't have a central scientific authority that can help resolve complicated debates. Instead, it lets the market decide, which often means that the bigger an organization's budget, the louder its voice. Nutritional science is especially hazy. Academic, government, nonprofit, and industry studies duke it out unrefereed in a Wild West atmosphere, made all the more confusing by the paid public relations gunslingers who fire diversionary shots into the crowd. These are not just the obvious food industry interests; the public needs to be wary of information coming from the pharmaceutical industry, some of the medical establishment, obesity experts, and the writers whose livelihoods depend on selling us diet books and programs. (Ironically, the only industry whose stake in our well-being matches our own appears to be the health and life insurance businesses, which stand to lose money from our ailments and untimely demises.)

For all of the aforementioned reasons, when presenting the current state of the science on sugar, it makes sense to rely on the staid World Health Organization (WHO), which has a careful and transparent process for developing, vetting, and getting nonprofit and industry feedback on its recommendations. The 2015 WHO sugar-intake guidelines do not address the fructose controversy, so we will ignore this until they do, but they do recommend that no more than 10 percent of total calories be from "free sugar." This category includes both added sugars and the natural sugars in fruit juice; it should also be noted that the clearest causal relationship the WHO found with sugar was with dental caries, not, as they are now called, noncommunicable diseases (NCDs) such as diabetes and heart disease. The case for an indirect relationship between sugar and NCDs is as follows: a diet high in added sugars makes it easier to gain weight, which can lead to obesity, and the obese are more likely to become diabetic. But even the link between added sugars and obesity isn't certain. When an Australian nutrition researcher at the University of Sydney, Jennie Brand Miller, who helped create the glycemic index, analyzed national data, she found that between 1995 and 2010–2011, intake of added sugars and sugar-sweetened beverages dropped by 10 percent in men, 20 percent in women, and even more in children, while obesity increased. This finding, so discordant with current public policy thinking, led to her being attacked—although ultimately forgiven—by other scholars.

We could have saved ourselves about half a century of research, but it appears that a calorie is a calorie, no matter what its source. A 2018 meta-analysis by researchers in Australia and China of twenty studies worldwide found that there is no difference between low-fat and high-fat diets in terms of weight gain in metabolically healthy overweight and obese people—and a mixed difference (part good, part bad) on blood lipids. Similarly, a 2017 Norwegian study found that nutrient proportion—high fat/low carb versus high carb/low fat—doesn't matter; you lose weight—and flubber—and prevent diabetes when you reduce caloric intake, period. There is no demon ingredient (or foodstuff, although best to limit sugary juices and sodas) responsible for our roly-poly selves—and, by extension, no evil food industry conspiracy to make us fat.

But if the devil isn't in the ingredients, perhaps it's in the additives? Again, widespread consumer alarm at laboratory-fabricated food add-ins is largely unwarranted. Food additives come in four functional categories: flavor, color, conditioning (to aid in processing or impart a specific characteristic), and preservatives. Other substances end up in small quantities in food as a result of agricultural processes, treatment to prolong the raw material's freshness and rid it of harmful microorganisms, and the mechanical and chemical techniques used to create edible products. The US Food and Drug Administration (FDA), the agency that oversees what companies can put into food, has a list of over three-thousand common additives.[5] When they are known or suspected to have negative health impacts, they are allowed only in minute quantities, a few parts per million. In addition, there are about one thousand or so additives that are Generally Recognized As Safe (GRAS) by the FDA and can be used without restriction.

The European Union has more stringent regulations than the United States, prohibiting a few more additives and requiring that labels state when products are made from genetically modified organisms (GMOs). But, on balance, these differences are small. "Most substances added to food [in the United States]—even ones with long chemical names—are safe," states the Center for Science in the Public Interest (CSPI) in a 2017 report on "clean" food labels. It goes on to note, however, that some are not, and others are poorly tested. But even with that caveat, there are only a handful of additives that are legal in the United States, but not in the European Union, noted below.

- **Azodicarbonamide (ADA)**: A softener and whitener for dough. Used mostly by quick-service restaurants such as sandwich and burger chains. During baking, it breaks down into chemicals that cause cancer in laboratory animals.

- **Butylated Hydroxyanisole (BHA) and Butylated Hydroxytoluene (BHT)**: Flavor enhancers and pre-servatives. Considered a likely carcinogen by the US government.

- **Brominated Vegetable Oil (BVO)**: Used to bind ingre-dients in citrus-flavored sodas and sports drinks. May contribute to body burden and affect memory, skin, and nerves.

---

5   https://www.fda.gov/food/food-additives-petitions/food-additive-status-list

- **Potassium Bromate**: A rising aid and whitener used in bread and other bakery products. A possible human carcinogen.

- **Red Food Dye No. 40 and Yellow Food Dyes No. 5 and No. 6**: Used in Europe with a warning label that may affect activity and attention of children.

The primary concern about this tiny list is decidedly old-school—cancer, with cognitive issues a distant second. None has been fingered as a magical obesity, cardiovascular, or metabolic-disease catalyst that somehow transforms the body into a fat-hoarding machine. (If you want to worry about what's in your food, maybe mull over some of the toxic byproducts of cooking, including acrylamide, PAHs (polycyclic aromatic hydrocarbons), and nitrosamines, and the short chains of synthetic polymers that migrate in from packaging.)

∽

For further proof that processed food, in and of itself, doesn't make you sick, let's cast our net a little wider—very wide, in fact—and look at a global analysis of food preparation habits. Handily, as part of another project, I conducted just such an analysis in 2018 with Robin Kanarek, then John Wade Professor of Psychology in the School of Arts and Sciences at Tufts University, and a small group of her students. We hunted down the original data for each country in a 2015 United Nations publication, *Time Use Across the World: Findings of a World Compilation of Time Use Surveys*, to see if we could put together a global portrait of how much time men and women dedicate to dinner. After some false starts and some errors, we were able to extract cooking and dish-doing data for fifty-two of the original sixty-five counties in the UN study, which I then correlated with WHO disease prevalence for the same countries and years. If industrial food is the root of all that ails you, and home food is a cure, we would expect to find that those places with the lowest rates of obesity and death from diabetes and heart disease would be where people cooked everything from scratch. Is that the case? Hardly.

DIABETES AND HEART DISEASE IN THE COUNTRIES WHERE WOMEN SPEND THE LEAST AMOUNT OF TIME ON FOOD-RELATED ACTIVITIES

Country	Women's Food Preparation Time (Minutes Daily)	Over-weight/ Obesity Rate (%)	Diabetes Death Rate (per 100,000)	Heart Disease Death Rate (per 100,000)	Smoking Prevalence	Inactivity Prevalence
US	49.2	64.8%	13.6	67.2	24.8	32.4
UK	54	60.6%	4.4	57.6	27.2	37.3
Sweden	57	53.9%	8	58.1	23.1	28.7
Denmark	58.2	53.3%	11	40.7	24.7	24.3
Thailand	60.3	26.7%	10.4	19.8	21.7	14.8
Finland	61.8	55.9%	4.4	88.1	23.5	23.5
NZ	62.3	62.7%	10.8	66.1	20.0	39.8
Norway	64.2	55.7%	6.5	45.9	26.9	25.8
Canada	65	61.2%	10.6	50.8	18.4	23.2
Austria	67.8	51.8%	14.6	70.3	35.7	23.8

Source: Data collection for all tables was done as a 2018 special project by the author with Brita Dawson, Rebecca Moragne, and Afua Ofori-Darko, students of Dr. Robin Kanarek, now Professor Emerita of Psychology at Tufts University. The food data was collected from the original sources—usually the national statistics bureau—for the 2015 *Time Use Across the World: Findings of a World Compilation of Time Use Surveys* by economist and statistician Jacques Charmes and published by the United Nations. Health data, with one exception, is from the World Health Organization. Smoking data comes from the World Bank.

If we choose the United States as an unhealthy baseline, with 64.8 percent of its adult population overweight or obese, a diabetes-related death rate of 13.6 per 100,000, a heart disease–related death rate of 67.2 per 100,000, and a 24.8 percent smoking prevalence during the study time period, which countries had even higher rates? Only two of the ten countries where women cook the least: Finland, which has a markedly slimmer overweight/obesity rate of 55.9 percent but similar smoking rate of 23.5 percent, a diabetes death rate of 4.4, and a heart disease death rate of 88.1. And Austria, which although slimmer still with an obesity rate of 51.8 percent, has a markedly higher smoking prevalence of 35.7 percent. The Austrians have a diabetes death rate of 14.6 per 100,000, and a heart disease death rate of 70.3.

DIABETES AND HEART DISEASE IN THE COUNTRIES WHERE WOMEN SPEND THE MOST AMOUNT OF TIME ON FOOD-RELATED ACTIVITIES

Country	Women's Food Preparation Time (Minutes Daily)	Over-weight/ Obesity Rate (%)	Diabetes Death Rate (per 100,000)	Heart Disease Death Rate (per 100,000)	Smoking Prevalence	Inactivity Prevalence
Algeria	168	57.4%	N/A	N/A	15.2	34.4
India	156	16.5%	N/A	N/A	14.3	13.4
Tunisia	155	57.8%	N/A	N/A	31.7	23.5
Pakistan	154.2	24.2%	N/A	N/A	21.3	26
Mauritius	154	29.3%	171.4	88.5	22.6	25.2
Albania	149.4	53.3%	0.3	60.0	31.2	N/A
Turkey	145.8	63.1%	25.2	63.8	30.8	32.8
Tanzania	144.8	23.8%	N/A	N/A	17.1	6.9
Serbia	138	54.3%	21.3	82.1	42.1	38.7
Romania	136.2	54.5%	6.6	21.3	32.8	25.3

Conversely, although half of the countries in which women cook the most are missing health data, three of the five that do have far worse cardiovascular and metabolic health indicators than the United States. In Mauritius, despite being relatively slim at a 29.3 percent overweight/obesity rate and a 22.6 percent smoking prevalence—similar to that of the United States, the diabetes death rate is a staggering 171.4 per 100,000, and the heart disease death rate is 88.5. In Turkey, where 63.1 percent of the adult population is overweight and obese and a considerable 30.8 percent smoke, death rates from diabetes and heart disease are 25.2 and 63.8, respectively. Serbia has similarly elevated statistics: 54.3 percent of adults are overweight or obese and 42.1 percent of those over fifteen years old smoke cigarettes; deaths from diabetes and heart disease are 21.3 and 82.1, respectively. In each of those countries, women dedicate between two and a quarter to two and a half hours a day to preparing food for their families.

Let's not be disingenuous. What's going on in these countries has little to do with whether they're ladling traditional dishes onto a plate or hitting the drive-through after work and everything to do with wealth. (And smoking!) In fact, a 2017 study by over two hundred medical researchers around the world and published in the *Journal of the American College of Cardiology* found that the strongest correlates with death rates from diabetes and heart disease are social and demographic: income per capita, educational attainment, and fertility rates. The scientists found that death rates from cardiovascular disease, especially from ischemic heart disease, were consistently higher in low and middle-income countries. They start to decline when nations reach a certain level of economic development. This is the exact opposite of the affluenza hypothesis that abundance and indolence breed lifestyle diseases.

Should food activists wish to continue to argue that from-scratch cooking has a salutary effect on health, let's examine the five countries with the highest rates of diabetes and heart disease–related deaths in the world. Are any of the countries where women spend the least amount of time in food preparation and cleanup, an advantage admittedly not only conferred by prepared and convenience food, but by the availability of moderately priced takeout (hello, Thailand) and more egalitarian arrangements when it comes to chores (hats off to the Scandinavians), among the least healthiest? Not a one.

LEAST HEALTHY COUNTRIES IN THE WORLD

Country	Over-weight/ Obesity Rate (%)	Diabetes Death Rate (per 100,000)	Heart Disease Death Rate (per 100,000)	Women's Food Prepara-tion Time (Minutes Daily)	Smoking Prevalence	Inactivity Preva-lence
FIVE COUNTRIES WITH HIGHEST DIABETES-RELATED DEATH RATES						
Mauritius	29.3%	171.4	----	154	22.6	25.2
Mexico	61.7%	91.6	----	103	17.1	26
South Africa	49.9%	64.7	----	87	21.0	46.9
Armenia	51.3%	37.2	----	115	29.3	N/A
Panama	55.2%	27.5	----	82	8.5	N/A
FIVE COUNTRIES WITH HIGHEST HEART-DISEASE-RELATED DEATH RATES						
Moldova	49.2%	----	371	121	23.9	12.3
Kyrgyz-stan	44.2%	----	332	102	26.6	13.3
Lithuania	57.6%	----	223	101	31.1	18.4
Armenia	51.3%	----	208	115	29.3	N/A
Latvia	55.8%	----	191	88	37.5	22

It doesn't seem that eating home-cooked meals makes much of a difference, at least when it comes to cardiovascular and metabolic diseases. In the five countries with the highest rates of diabetes-related deaths—Mauritius, Mexico, South Africa, Armenia, and Panama, women cook from a low of 82 minutes per day in Panama to a high of 154 in Mauritius. Similarly, in the five countries with the highest rates of heart disease–related deaths—Moldova, Kyrgyzstan, Lithuania, Armenia, and Latvia, women hunker down over their ovens for a low of 88 minutes in Latvia to a high of 121 minutes in Moldova. No one is any better for it for the simple reasons that people get fat when they eat more calories than they burn, no matter what the macronutrient content of the food and if it was prepared in a home kitchen or on a factory floor, and diet isn't the most important factor contributing to their health.

∞

I don't know about you, but there are a lot of things that keep me up at night: paying the bills, random acts of violence and terrorism, finding my next consulting job, paying for college, school shootings, the rise of American nationalism, growing income disparity, homelessness, saving for retirement, being displaced from my consulting job by artificial intelligence, fire, climate change, the next pandemic, financial market meltdowns, missing writing deadlines, that my husband or I will accidentally mow down a bicyclist and lose our house and our meager savings in a lawsuit, losing our health insurance, failing. It's fair to say that the world is in one of its more precarious moments and in the face of that instability, most of us have a single impulse: hide.

And what more soothing place to retreat to than the details of a complicated diet? My brother omits fat from his, swapping in liquid egg whites and skinny cheeses and eating chicken, chicken, chicken. Our friends Mira and Geoff read *Grain Belly* and are no longer consuming carbohydrates. (I refrain from pointing out that they are no longer eating *simple* carbohydrates; vegetables have plenty of complex ones.) They have lost weight, and they feel great! When they were eating wheat, their minds just felt so clouded. Their contribution to our potluck—a delicious roast cauliflower with Indian spices and uncooked, sugar-free butter-and-cocoa cookies. My brother-in-law, and now my sister, are adherents of intermittent fasting, which they believe amps up their insulin sensitivity, preventing diabetes. (I'm guessing having two super hangry owners has made the work environment in their small architecture business delightful.) My cousin NayNay—understandably careful after a bout with cancer—and friend Diana, both longtime committed vegans, have gone the extra mile and followed the *New York Times* one-month sugar detox. Now that they are no longer being poisoned by sweetness, whole foods taste so much better. And their blood sugar levels are no longer constantly spiking, keeping them on a Zen-like keel throughout the day.

The friends and relatives I've had that have lost weight/gained energy/improved their mood/cleared their skin by adhering to, variously, gluten-free, keto, vegan, high-protein, and other nutritional plans are too numerous to count. Substitute some religious terminology for the foodstuffs they abstain from and you've got yourself a conversion experience: after sinning by huffing bread and rice, mainlining fried and fatty foods, or gorging themselves on cake and candy, the individual is enlightened by one of the dozen or so food gurus—the almost all-white, all-male pantheon includes Michael Pollan (eat only whole foods), Robert Lustig (no sugar), Gary Taubes (no sugar), William Davis (no gluten), Jason Fung (intermittent fasting; at least he's Asian—and Canadian), and Robert Atkins (no carbs; high fat and protein), each of whom advocates their particular brand of wellness philosophy. After following strict rules, the person is saved. This sort of asceticism is nothing new: the spiritual glow one gets from self-denial is part and parcel of all major world religions, from Christianity and Judaism to Buddhism and Islam. But what is unique—at least in this day and age; the ancient Greeks practiced it as part of athletic training—is its cooption for secular purposes and downgrading of the quest for spiritual transcendence to mere physical well-being.

Several years ago, I abruptly lost hearing in the upper ranges in both ears. I saw an otolaryngologist; a radiologist; a neurologist; two neurotologists, specialists in the neurology of the inner ear; and got tested up the wazoo (short list: Lyme disease, diabetes, syphilis, HIV/AIDS, lupus, rheumatoid arthritis, sarcoidosis, allergies), but no one could figure out what was wrong with me. So I did what we all do in times of great stress, I put my faith in a higher power—the internet. If I googled long enough and with the exact right combination of search terms, I would magically discover my diagnosis, and, with luck, the cure. Which is why from Friday, October 28, 2011, 9:38 A.M. ET, the moment I read about "secondary endolymphatic hydrops," in which an increased volume of inner ear fluid presses on the cochlea and (balm to my drug-fearing soul), which can be controlled with a special diet, I decided to stop eating salt and sugar—ruling out any kind of processed food.

The special diet didn't restore my hearing, but following it for a month opened my eyes to how pervasive industrial food really is. I'm a relatively healthy eater, although under duress I'll concede that only a third of my calories come from whole or from-scratch food and the other two-thirds from sweets and treats (chocolate, ice cream, crackers, chips, olives, cheese) or the stuff that in a distant time or place would be relegated to the family pig—pizza crusts; half-eaten sandwiches; sad, little, ketchup-dabbed chicken nuggets. By noon of my first day on the regime, I was already panicked. What would I eat? I swung open the refrigerator and gazed longingly inside. Vast swaths of edibles, all off limits: frozen pizza, pot stickers, deli meats, cheese, condiments, peanut butter, jam and jelly, pickles. I slid open the vegetable compartment—lettuce, carrots, celery. A start. But what about the substance? A sprinkling of unsalted sunflower seeds? My stomach growled. How about an egg, crisply fried in a pool of butter? Scratch that, the butter has salt. Oh dear. I was going to be hungry. Very, very hungry. Over the course of that month, I didn't lose weight, have more energy, or feel happier. In fact, I felt grumpy, tired, and deprived.

The experts are still arguing about the causes of lifestyle diseases. The most circumspect scientists say their origins are multifactorial and include access to medicine and medical interventions, smoking, alcohol, diet, and physical activity. But this is a cop-out. It may cover your posterior when it comes to medical malpractice, but the world has an urgent need for more exact information so that it can improve quality of life and reduce premature death for millions. Can't we assign a weight to how much each of these factors contributes? (Smoking's devastating influence is, after decades of disinformation from the tobacco industry, finally irrefutable, so on that factor, at least, discussion closed.)

For example, it's clear that access to medical care is probably the single most important thing we can do to save lives. While the countries with the highest rates of diabetes and heart disease rates are all over the map when it comes to obesity, smoking, and physical activity, they are unified by one thing: their lack of infrastructure, including health-care systems. Tragically, we don't even need to point to these low and middle-income illustrations; we can just compare the United States to its two closest peers, Canada and the United Kingdom. Despite having similar economies and cultures, the United States has a higher death rate for both diabetes and heart disease. (It should be noted that Brits have higher rates of smoking and inactivity than Americans, while Canadians have less.) What's one of the biggest differences among the three English-speaking nations? The United States has no national health system, meaning that some Americans have no insurance and others are footing mind-bogglingly large bills for hospitalizations and medications. The result, especially when combined with disparate rates of noncommunicable diseases for those with low incomes and communities of color, led to the shocking spectacle of one of the wealthiest countries in the world having the most deaths during the COVID-19 pandemic.

During the late twentieth and early twenty-first centuries, Hippocrates's famous (and apparently misquoted) dictum, "Let food be thy medicine, and medicine be thy food," has been tossed about like rice at a wedding. But no one has been able to prove it. Yet we spend countless hours and billions of dollars on weight loss schemes or special nutrition. If a "good diet" is not the powerful panacea people imagine—an inviting illusion, because who doesn't enjoy thinking about food and eating it?—then we are wasting vast amounts of resources and endangering lives. A December 2019 PubMed search for the terms *diet, nutrition,* and *food,* along with *cardiovascular, diabetes, heart disease,* and *obesity* yielded 303,371 results. A search of three terms related to physical activity and the lifestyle diseases turns up about half that, 189,663; smoking, 102,951; and alcohol, 38,620. But a search for healthcare access and the same terms, just 5,501.

One of my favorite thought experiments is to imagine I'm viewing my family from afar, like a child peeping in through the roof of a dollhouse. Since Rafi and I work from home, that looks something like this: significant other sits for hours on end in an office chair, then eats, and reclines for several more hours on a couch. Then he goes to bed. This may be punctuated by driving the car to drop off or pick up a teenager, a trip to the supermarket or Home Depot, gardening or home repairs, or a photography shoot. (Not to cast stones; my day is about the same, but I do run faithfully for forty minutes to an hour.) My two youngest daughters' activity logs aren't much better. Both practice a seasonal, travel-team sport—soccer and gymnastics—with plenty of aerobic conditioning, but it's another story during the off months. They take the bus to school, maybe do an extracurricular activity, and take the bus home (or more often, plead for a ride). In the house, they sit at their desks, lie on their beds, sit at the counter, and lie on the sofa. For all of us, most of these activities take place within inches or feet of a screen-based electronic device. Tell me your day is any different.

Over the early to mid-twentieth century, the automobile, factory mechanization, and domestic appliances reduced the amount of time people spent moving their bodies. But Americans truly settled into their stationary ways with the arrival of the television. By 1970, 95 percent of homes had a set and the average person sat transfixed by it for six hours daily, according to the Statistical Abstracts of the United States (SAUS). Still, because programming could only be watched at certain hours and channels were few, adults still did other recreational activities—bowling, knitting, and reading—and children still played outside, as we did in my neighborhood in the mid-1970s. (Although I remember some long, open-mouthed, television-viewing sessions, mostly cartoons.) Unfortunately, this period was relatively idyllic compared to the present era.

Since the mid-1970s, our love affair with screens has grown at warp speed. Without diminishing our ardor for television, the consumption of which rose to over seven hours daily in 1990 (SAUS), electronic entertainment options exploded. In 1975 the video game *Pong*, played through a console attached to the TV, was released. Its raging success spawned an industry that today shows no sign of abating. But prying controllers, and later joysticks, out of the hands of frenzied adolescents would be fruitless. Other electronic toys were popping up like prairie dogs. In the mid- to late 1970s, home video recorders (VCRs) began to allow people to watch feature-length movies in their own homes. In the same period, the very first personal computers, the clunky Commodore PET and the Apple II, began to be sold in tech centers across the nation—by 1984, 8.2 percent of homes had a computer, according to the US Census. That same year, the Cable Act removed regulatory barriers from cable television, and channels proliferated; some experimented with deliberately provocative talk shows, a format that stuck; these broadcast shoutfests are now as mainstream as the nightly news once was. (Let's not forget MTV, whose three-minute music videos foreshadowed YouTube's commitment-averse format, which rarely lasts for more than ten minutes.) And we haven't yet arrived at the biggest transformations—and continual captors of our attention—the World Wide Web (1991) and smartphones (technically IBM in 1992, but come on, the 2007 iPhone) that could do it all: telephone and text, take pictures and video, play music, and surf the by now omnipresent internet.

This has given rise to a new phenomenon: multiscreening. The media-tracking and analysis company Nielsen gleefully asks in a December 2018 newsletter post: "With all of this technology at consumers' literal fingertips, which of these platforms are they focused on? The answer, in short, is pretty much all of them." This adds up to about ten and a half hours a day that adults spend on TVs, TVs and connected devices, and radio and digital platforms (computer, smartphones, and tablets). That's a hell of a lot of hours! In fact, even if people sleep only six hours a night, this leaves a mere seven and a half hours in which to cram all other activities, including grooming, eating, housework, childcare, errands, and, oh yes, work. So it shouldn't be a revelation that a full 80 percent of Americans do no exercise or recreational sports at all, according to the American Time Use Survey (ATUS). That omission is compounded by the reverential stillness most of us evince when interacting with our beloved apparatuses. We are now more immobile than ever before in human history.

New research shows the damaging effects of sedentarism, sitting or lying for long periods of time. It is slowly being acknowledged as as much (or even more) of a risk factor as poor diet in obesity and illness. Insufficient physical activity is highly correlated with diabetes, heart disease, high blood pressure, and high cholesterol, risks that are exacerbated when combined with a regular caloric surfeit (i.e., weight gain). Over the past two decades, for the first time ever, the rate of all-cause mortality in the United States has increased for adults under the age of sixty-five. In addition to the recent spike in deaths because of the COVID-19 pandemic, much of this comes from the manyfold increase in drug overdoses from opioids; Virginia Commonwealth University School of Medicine researchers calculate some forty-one thousand additional lost lives. But deaths linked to organ system diseases are also up by thirty thousand, among them five thousand from hypertension-related illnesses.

In the past seventy years, US death rates for heart disease and stroke have improved dramatically, thanks to lower smoking rates and improved—and improved access to—medical prevention and treatment. In 1950 the death rates per 100,000 for heart disease and stroke were 588.8 and 180.7, respectively; today they are 165.0 and 37.6 (although, as noted before, these rates are higher than those of our peer countries.) We have not made such progress on metabolic diseases—which are, significantly, the ones most sensitive to obesity; the needle has only nudged from 23.1 in 1950 to 21.5 in 2017.

What's the answer?

∽

My parents' approaches to caring for their bodies were polar opposites.

As a young man, addled by Beatnik troubadours wailing "500 Miles" and "Freight Train," my father rode the rails. On one trip, he crossed the border to Mexico, probably through El Paso, and found himself walking the line at night after an evening at the cantina. In the dark, he fell off a trestle over a gully, and passed out. He woke up the next morning splayed over a rock and in pain. After that, his back bothered him for the rest of his life. In the late 1960s, when he had a young family and was working as a schoolteacher in a small Vermont town, he took up jogging to cope with the constant discomfort. This at the time unheard-of practice elicited crowds of gawking teenagers (his students) and smartass comments from adults such as "What are you running from? Your wife?" But the sport strengthened my father's back muscles and reduced his spasms. Running six, eight, ten miles a day became his habit for the next forty years.

My mother, on the other hand, had been a butterball as a young girl, and while she blossomed into a slim young woman with a serene gaze and incandescent smile, she waged a battle with her weight her entire adult life. Although she got some exercise through housework and gardening, her principle tool was diet. There were a couple intense affairs with Weight Watchers and "health food" a la Francis Moore Lappe (oh sunflower-seed-studded, honey-sweetened, whole wheat cookies of my youth, I remember you still and shudder), but mostly her approach was to strip any enjoyment from the food. Small, lean, overcooked pieces of chicken or hamburger, devoid of sauce. Plain, steamed broccoli, squash, or carrots. Rice and potatoes, unsullied by even a grain of salt. Despite her punitive approach to victualing, she still gained weight, at one point topping two hundred pounds.

I often daydream about making a poster—trigger alert—featuring the two standing side by side naked: my father lean, well-muscled, and vibrant (although he died relatively young of pancreatic cancer); my mother bent, heavy, and tired. She was a disease magnet, starting in her thirties with a brain tumor and then moving to a stroke, rheumatoid arthritis, and Parkinson's, all underlain by high blood pressure, high cholesterol, and atherosclerosis. Her joints hurt, she could hardly walk, and, during her last five years, lived confined to her bedroom and our dining room. "Exercises," it would say under my father. "Doesn't," under my mother.

Long-distance runners, as their friends and families know all too well, love to humblebrag about their amped-up metabolisms. "I eat anything I want," they say, sitting across the table from you wolfing down wedges of cake, bowls of pasta, and bags of chips with a winsome smile on their gaunt-cheeked faces. "And I never gain weight!" (Well, of course not, you ninny, you have one thousand additional calories above baseline to play with.) But while they may like to coyly flaunt their enormous appetites and slim physiques, it's worthwhile to note that no matter what the content of their plates, they almost never suffer from type 2 diabetes, prediabetes/metabolic syndrome, high cholesterol, high blood pressure, and atherosclerosis. While some runners follow rigorous training diets, others do not. If unhealthy food really were the cause of so many illnesses, at least some of these fitness devotees would suffer from them, too. But they don't.

This is a clue.

It's not our food that's making us sick, but the lack of something endurance athletes have in spades: daily metabolic workouts in which the body must gear up to supply energy at a very high rate. Aerobic exercise shifts the body from its sedentary holding pattern in which its two fuels, glucose and fatty acids, enter into cells in their proportion in the bloodstream, to full-steam-ahead operations with a circulation up to four times faster (in non-athletes) and a calorie-burn rate that is four to eight times faster than sitting. In this state, the immense energy needs of heart and muscles are prioritized, and instead of leaving it up to chance, the body tailors the blood's nutrient mix to meet them. Rather than allow molecules to wash through their outer membranes according to the last meal or their fasting-state proportion, cells select which type of energy to consume and send signals so that the bloodstream delivers exactly that. Over time, this process remakes the cardiovascular system and key metabolic pathways, imparting good health.

While there have been some improvements, the overall exercise picture is bleak. CDC data on physical activity in the past decades shows
that in 1998, just 14.3 percent of adults met minimum requirements for
both aerobic and strengthening activity; by 2017, that had increased to
24.5. But, unfortunately, leisure-time exercise does not compensate for
the well-documented loss of activity in other realms of life: work, in
which physical occupations have dropped by 83 percent between 1950
and 2000, and transportation, in which the people who walk to work or
for errands has declined by 71 percent in the same time period, according
to researchers at the Saint Louis University School of Public Health.
Nationally recognized exercise researchers Frank W. Booth and P. Darrell
Neufer, in a 2005 article in *American Scientist* argue, "Our underuse of
skeletal muscle may play an under-recognized role in the rise of chronic
disease as a cause of modern mortality."

I don't eat a family-sized bag of Nacho Doritos every day anymore,
although I enjoy potato chips, candy, desserts, and alcohol in modera-
tion. Aside from crackers and cheese, I don't eat a lot of heavily processed
foods. But I don't bat an eye when my husband pops a frozen dinner into
the microwave or when my daughter cooks up a package of ramen. (Okay,
I do bat an eye; those things are sodium bombs.) I avail myself freely of
prepared items such as tomato sauce, pasta, boxed pilafs and mixed rices,
canned beans and tuna, all kinds of sauces and condiments, frozen pizza,
frozen vegetables and fruits, ice cream and cookies, greens and salads in
a bag, and instant coffee. I'm not fat, and neither is any member of my
family, although Rafi, now in his fifth decade, sports what he calls *buena
vida* around the middle. Not only that, I'm extraordinarily healthy for
my age, or any age, with a low pulse, good blood pressure, and perfect
cholesterol (and my MS has been dormant for three decades). This has
nothing to do with what I eat—or don't—and everything to do with the
four miles I run every day.

4

Meaty Mice and the Men and Women Who Overfeed Them

It had been a good trip. We stayed with our friends, Ariana and Beto, whom Rafi had met thirty years ago at La Universidad de la Habana. Every day, we explored a new section of Miami—Buena Vista, Design District, Little Havana, Miami Beach, and Wynwood, Rafi with his camera—he planned to start a new travel-oriented line of his architectural photography business, and me with the girls, sightseeing, trinket-shopping, and snacking. At night, we went out for dinner and then hung out in our hosts' screened-in patio, talking until late. We'd done a weekend trip to Naples, where the seven of us spent two days stretched out on perfect white beaches. (Okay, I walked; sunbathing isn't my thing.) That morning, we'd gotten up at 5:00 A.M., driven our over-priced rental to Fort Lauderdale, and boarded our 8:00 A.M., Sunday Spirit Airline flight to Boston. I reclined in my seat and closed my eyes. My Cuban-born husband had gotten his infusion of midwinter warmth. My kids had bonded with Ariana and Beto's son, Emanuel, and been exposed to their paternal culture. And I had a chance to breathe and do what I most like, wander—in my daily runs, in my walks around the city, and in my mind, daydreaming about the light, vegetation, architecture, and people. It was February 19, 2020, and it would be our last normal day for the next two years.

I had already had inklings from my public health work—I'd even mentally assessed our travel risk of contracting the novel coronavirus that had appeared in China and was starting to sprout up in other places around the globe: low. It had floated into my head a couple times—especially at the Presidents' Day mob at the Miami Museum of Science, where I'd gone to give a talk on processed foods and the military to an audience whose average age was probably four. (They asked very incisive questions: "Is it bad to eat like soldiers? Can I have these M&Ms?") A week after our return, the girls' school sent out the first ominous/reassuring message urging us to "please remember that one reason this virus has been so devastating is that it is a new virus, and there is therefore no vaccine to help prevent its spread. Like the flu, COVID-19 can make people very sick, but most people recover fully." Two weeks later, the school system halted in-person classes and condemned students to study remotely indefinitely.

At our house, this ushered in an abrupt change in routines. Not for Rafi and me, who are both mostly glued to our chairs in our basement offices, pleasantly cool in summer and, at least mine, which is in the old part of the house, noticeably dank in the winter. But suddenly our two high-flying daughters were grounded. Gabriela, seventeen, went from weeks that included taking the train downtown a couple afternoons to volunteer in an organization that gave free legal services for immigration, housing, and occupational issues; working shifts at a local supermarket; a Saturday enrichment program; and weekend excursions and sleepovers with friends to . . . nothing. Mariela, sixteen, went from several after-school STEM programs, evening gymnastics practices, and weekend activities like hackathons and Splashes to . . . nothing. The school moved session start times to midmorning and even noon. Soon both girls were staying up all night, doing their online classes from bed, then hiding in their messy rooms until Rafi and I had gone upstairs to sleep. "I think it's a need for privacy," I told him. "They're carving out their own world at night because we are all here 24/7 and can't go anyplace."

Around 11:30 P.M., when the coast was clear, they ventured out of their attic lairs. I would hear music, voices, and laughter and smell cooking—black beans and yellow rice, chicken nuggets and french fries, bacon, macaroni and cheese, smoothies, and ramen, ramen, ramen. In the morning when I came down, the counters were littered with half-eaten plates of food and packaging, the stovetop was a jumble of dirty pots and pans, the sink was piled high with dishes, and the trash overflowing, spreading old coffee grounds and banana peels in a splash pattern that even extended through the ragged hole I'd noticed in the plywood separating the dishwasher from the sink drain. I would sigh and start cleaning up. It wasn't the way I wanted to start the day, but I sensed that underneath their reversed daily rhythms was fear—their lives had been overturned and the grown-ups had no answers. Whatever comfort their nocturnal meals gave them, I did not want to deprive them of it.

A few months into lockdown, we were already yearning to escape. After a frightening period in which diagnoses climbed daily, hospitals filled to capacity, and morgues were supplemented with refrigerated containers, case numbers began declining. This hopeful sign was echoed by nature. It was May, and, heedless of what was happening in the human realm, the world was awash in flowers and tender green leaves. For years, our extended family had convened in Vermont on Memorial Day to celebrate my mother's birthday. She was no longer here. And we couldn't mingle with people from another household for fear of infecting one another. But Rafi, Mariela, and I decided to go up anyway. We arrived, made dinner with the groceries we'd brought with us from Boston, and settled into a rollicking game of Scrabble with a 1950s set missing numerous letters. As usual, we'd gotten into an unspoken contest to see who could fool the others with the most preposterous invented word, making for a lot of banter and sidelong glances to see if anyone's poker face would crack. Around 11:30 P.M., my telephone rang. Gabi, who'd informed us she no longer enjoyed the country and begged to be left in the house alone for the first time. Probably scared.

"Mami! Papi! There's a rat in the living room!"

"Are you sure?"

"It's staring at me!"

Phone in hand, she ran the two flights upstairs to her bedroom, while we tried to coach her on crisis-management skills from afar. After twenty minutes, she seemed to calm down, and we hung up. But the festive mood had evaporated. We climbed into bed, quietly staring into our phones. I didn't say anything and neither did Rafi, but I knew we were both googling rats. We turned out the lights, and were jolted by another call.

"Mami, Papi, they're trying to get into my room. I hear gnawing."

"They're Norway rats," I told her, putting my newly gleaned information to use. "They are burrowers and I'm sure they got in through the basement. I doubt they would go up to the attic—there's no food there." Well, I thought, but didn't say, except for the half-eaten bowls of noodles, partially consumed bags of chips, and open boxes of crackers under Mariela's bed.

"If you're really scared, I can call Miriam and ask if you can sleep there."

"No, it's okay. I'll be all right."

Suddenly, evidence of the rats was everywhere. Once we got home, I pulled out the trash and recycling baskets from under the sink. The ragged hole in the plywood separator from the dishwasher was even bigger—and obviously a rodent entrance and exit. How had I not realized it? I thought back to the day a month before when the double mousetrap (we've peacefully coexisted with their small cousins for years) had caught two extraordinarily plump specimens, which Rafi proudly waved at me. "Wow," I said. "Even their tails are fat." Now I saw a vision of a mama rat proudly leading her babies on their first foraging trip. Bang. Bang.

Nervous about their presence, I forewent the music I habitually played while I worked. Scuffle, scuffle, scuffle. Gnaw, gnaw, gnaw. The rats' footsteps seemed to patter over my head—and in the dropped ceiling of my office, the one filled with improperly grounded wiring. The gnawing was in the ceiling of our electrical room, roughly under the stove. Rafi and I dashed to the shed and rolled out the bins—their bottom edges were so chewed they looked like plastic lace—to inspect the old fieldstone foundation. It was riddled with holes. Suddenly, I could picture their entire domain. It extended from the shed under the front porch where we kept our trash receptacles, through the closet where I keep cleaning and paper supplies, across my office ceiling, to emerge—oh, the folly of incuriosity—under the dishwasher, which had stopped working a few months ago, and the stove, which just recently had refused to turn on. Even though our 1870s Victorian house has three stories and two finished basement rooms, in their abode, everything was on the same plane. "It's like the rats have their own private ranch house inside our house," I said to Rafi. And they were as fiercely attached to it as we were to ours. They bustled about with impunity—back and forth to the food stores and inside the walls. I knocked. They ignored me. I knocked again. They continued to ignore me. We'd been invaded.

They were not only unafraid; they weren't about to cede an inch. I felt overwhelmed and helpless. Luckily, these were exactly the circumstances in which Rafi had grown up. Trying to get just about anything done in a communist dictatorship had taught him to be wily, persistent, and patient. His first step was an Amazon spending spree: daily packages arrived with an infinite variety of traps, from the Victor No-Touch No-See Electronic and Cat Sense Covered to glue pans. He became obsessed with a remote corner of YouTube dedicated to DIY rat-catching, and, with some items from Staples, built several plastic storage box–based contraptions. Particularly notable was the trapdoor model, which the rat accessed by climbing along a tube and then, after being lured out onto the top of the box by a trail of seeds and peanut butter, suddenly fell through a trapdoor in the middle. I also admired the walk-the-plank version, in which the rat inched along a board toward an edible prize until the plank suddenly gave way under its weight, plunging it into the water below. Rafi set them out and instructed us not to move them. "Rats are cautious," he told us. "They won't touch it at first. We need to let them explore, and then once they let their guard down . . . bam!" Needless to say, our rats were not fooled. By early summer, they had become so brazen that they began an extensive remodel, making new and better passageways to access our kitchen. I heard them gnawing in the walls, scurrying across my office ceiling, and setting in like dental jackhammers in the kitchen floor under the stove. I took to pounding on the wall with a broomstick for minutes at a time. They didn't miss a beat with their incessant mastication of our beams, studs, floorboards, drywall, plaster, and wiring. On my birthday in July, we invited family for a masked meal on our deck. When I went into the kitchen to throw out the disposable hors d'oeuvre plates and bring out the main course—yes, I make and serve my own birthday meals—I saw a long tail plunge into the trash where my hand had just been. I stifled a scream and returned outside as if nothing had happened. Our house-keeping is the subject of good-natured jibes—my brother-in-law, who's 6'3", ostentatiously runs his forefinger over our doorjambs and examines it with dismay; my sister gets out a dish towel and polishes our glasses before serving herself a drink. But what would they say if they knew our house was teeming with large, sleek, and aggressive rats? I kept quiet and served the pesto and Cuban chicken.

While catching our unwanted rodent guests remained elusive, Rafi was more successful at exclusion, one of the critical legs of rat control. On multiple occasions, he slowly circled the house with a bucket of quick-dry cement, slapping it into any hole he found bigger than a dime between the ground and three feet up, where the asbestos shingles begin. Although I'd been avoiding it, he insisted I come into the shed under the porch with him to show me his handiwork: the repair was so extensive that the previously rough and rathole-riddled old fieldstone with its dry mortar was now as smooth as a poured-concrete wall. A few days later, we smelled something awful. It faded, and then a new awful smell appeared. The great die-off had begun. A few weeks later, the sounds from inside the framework of our house had quieted. Not only that, for the first time in over a decade, there was no sign of the mice that drag away the crumbs from under our toaster and nibble the crispy particles that surround our burners. Rafi had won!

∞

Much to our annoyance, mice and rats have inhabited human settlements since we first began storing food—in fact, the genus name *mus* means "to steal" in Sanskrit. Until recently, this relationship was commensal: they benefited, we didn't, but weren't harmed. Pet versions of the animals, often unusually colored, were kept as early as China's Han Dynasty (206 B.C.E.–220 C.E.), and in the nineteenth century, "fancy mice" became a British, and then an American, fad. The first "fancy rats" appeared a little earlier and have a bloodthirsty origin. They were the lucky beauties kept aside by rat catchers from the thousands they caught for rat-baiting, a sport in which dogs competed to kill the most rats in a small pit. After this, "women are largely cross-breeding them kind of intuitively," explains Richard Pell, the director of the Center for PostNatural History in Pittsburg, Pennsylvania. "This is pre-Mendel, pre-Darwin, in a lot of cases. The mechanisms aren't well understood, but the outcomes are. You know, you're getting . . . different patterns in the fur, and different colors that don't exist in nature." Seeking substitutes for the cute puppies and bunnies that tended to get antivivisectionists all apoplectic—and to this day, the fallback figureheads for groups such as People for the Ethical Treatment of Animals (PETA), early twentieth-century scientists turned to these pedigreed breeds. After all, who cared what happened to animals that have always been considered vermin? (Americans dedicate some $800 million a year to their elimination, according to *Pest Control Technology* magazine's annual report.) It was thus that humankind finally domesticated rats and mice, says Pell—as "furry test tubes."

Today medical research advances on billions of tiny rodent paws (which, while not as dexterous as human hands, are excellent for climbing and holding food). According to the American Anti-Vivisection Society, 93 percent of all biomedical studies are done on rats and mice—but no one knows exactly how many. This ignorance is by design: in 2002, after intense lobbying by the National Association for Biomedical Research, the Animal Welfare Act, which regulates the treatment of laboratory animals, was amended to exclude rats, mice, and birds because, it was claimed, overseeing their well-being would be too expensive. (The National Institutes of Health's regulations do cover mice and rats, but unlike the US Department of Agriculture, they don't do annual inspections. Europe and Canada both protect and do as-warranted inspections of rodents.) "Anecdotally, anybody who does the kind of work I've done knows that there are tons more mice and rats than there used to be in the late eighties," says Larry Carbone, a veterinarian who has specialized in laboratory animal care for forty years and wrote the 2004 book *What Animals Want: Expertise and Advocacy in Laboratory Animal Welfare Policy.* "So everybody knows, though nobody has really quite documented, that making transgenic mice, inventing transgenic mice, led to skyrocketing increases in mice numbers." Absent official data, in 2021 Carbone estimated that 111 million mice and rats are subjects of experiments in the United States every year: "Off the cuff, I'd say probably a third are genetically modified animals." One of the most common uses is in studies of obesity, diabetes, cardiovascular disease, and metabolic illnesses. A search on PubMed with those terms and *rat* turns up 1.3 million studies and is 70 percent of all research that mentions the word *rat*. Search them with *mice*, and there are 1.2 million results, 66 percent of all items with the term *mice*.

Some of these studies are from the lab directed by Laurie J. Goodyear, a cell biologist and exercise physiologist in the Integrative Physiology and Metabolism Section at Joslin Diabetes Center in Boston. Goodyear is a direct woman with straight, strawberry-blonde hair and a pedometer permanently affixed to her hip. At the end of the workday, if the readout hasn't reached ten thousand steps, she paces the halls until it does. She also swims, plays soccer, jogs, and lifts weights. She is a workout fanatic because of her decades of research, which have shown her aerobic exercise is the best way to prevent and control type 2 diabetes, bar none. After some running-based bonding—mileage, cross-training, and injuries, we talk about her work—and her mice. I first contacted her after reading about her early and important study on Sprague-Dawley rats—the red-eyed, white-furred cuties most people picture when you say "laboratory animal"—showing that exercise causes glucose to enter cells even without being triggered by insulin. In that study, nineteen male rats were kept in a 73.4 degree Fahrenheit room for four days, eating and drinking to their hearts' content. Then, nine of the animals were removed and made to run on a treadmill for an hour and twenty minutes, while their control group peers lounged about their cages doing nothing. Immediately afterward, all the rats were killed with a blow to the head and their muscle tissue removed for analysis. Goodyear and her colleagues found that the amount of glucose transporter four (GLUT4), one of a family of a dozen or so proteins around the body that usher glucose into cells, was 45 percent higher in the exercised rats than in the controls. "The present study demonstrates that exercise causes a redistribution of glucose transporters from an intracellular microsomal pool to the plasma membrane. . . . Our findings suggested that exercise and insulin stimulate the same transport system."[6]

This was a huge breakthrough. Until then, scientists had believed that the only way to get GLUT4 to move to the skeletal muscle cell membrane was when insulin attached to membrane, setting off a chain reaction that eventually reached and liberated the GLUT4 proteins from their nearby storage compartments. (Insulin is a hormone released by the pancreas when blood sugar levels are high; it tells skeletal muscle, heart, liver, and fat cells to take in glucose.) But here was proof that exercise tripped a second signaling pathway that also caused GLUT4 to activate glucose uptake. For people with either type 1 or type 2 diabetes, knowing that exercise could help them regulate blood sugar, even without insulin, gave them a powerful new tool for managing and, in the case of lifestyle-related diabetes, preventing the disease.

Before talking with Goodyear, I'd watched an online video in which she talked about some of her later experiments on mouse muscles so I knew a little about how she got her tiny subjects to work out. "We have a rodent treadmill. . . . And these can be for training studies, chronic exercise, or they can be used for acute studies. We can actually do studies in the lab of chronic exercise where we put animals in wheel tables and they will voluntarily exercise, which is a much better way to exercise animals than treadmill running [forced by electric shocks]. . . . How much will a typical gray mouse this long exercise in one day? . . . Six miles a day, with legs this long!"[7] As excited as I was about talking with Goodyear about one of the hidden mechanisms by which physical activity opens up a whole new layer of cellular and molecular processes, my mind snagged on that little, gray mouse indefatigably running.

---

6 Laurie J. Goodyear, Michael F. Hirshman, and Edward S. Horton, "Exercise-Induced Translocation of Skeletal Muscle Glucose Transporters," *American Journal of Physiology* 261, no. 6 (1991): E798–79.

7 https://www.youtube.com/watch?v=5WHKZrGaSJo, around minute 8:30.

I ask Goodyear if the mice in her lab, or at Harvard in general, have wheels in their cages to accommodate this powerful urge to run. No, she tells me, unless physical activity is part of the experimental protocol. And could you even compare an animal that is constantly in motion to one, like us, that intersperses a few periods of activity with long rests? Goodyear concurs that this is a basic difference between mice and humans and, for that matter, mice and rats, who are almost as exertion-averse as we are. "If you have a mouse, and it does a bout of exercise, and then you measure their blood glucose level, or other indicators of their glucose homeostasis, they're not affected as much by exercise . . . because they're just doing that all the time anyway," says Goodyear. But, she is quick to add, "In some ways, yeah, mice aren't good models, but in other ways, they are very good. Because certainly, you know, things that we, if we look at the muscle of a mouse that exercises and compare it to the muscle of a human that we exercise, it's pretty much always the same responses."

∽

The catapulting of the mouse from household nuisance to the preferred in vivo research fodder for the world's scientific laboratories is the work of one man: Clarence Cook Little (1888–1971), a Harvard-trained geneticist whose career included stints as the eugenics-espousing president of the University of Michigan and head of the Tobacco Industry Research Committee, the organization responsible for obfuscating the public with confusing and contradictory smoking studies. It started with Abbie Lathrop (1868–1918), a Massachusetts entrepreneur whose talent for breeding pet rodents—she kept as many as eleven thousand on her farm—eventually landed her a gig providing mice, rats, and guinea pigs to clients such as the US government and Harvard University. Little, a young scientist in Harvard's Bussey Institute for Research in Applied Biology, took Lathop's work and ran with it, creating Black 6, a new substrain of inbred mice—the result of a long series of incestuous matings between parents and children or between siblings—from one of hers. "He had read Mendel's papers, [and he knew that] what is true for the pea plant is true for everything else," says Pell. "He saw an opportunity there to create inbred research models so that people could be doing genetics research on essentially the same platform. Because they wanted to have repeatable results. And how do you have repeatable results, if everyone's mice are a little different? You needed to have a single source, where you could say all of these are essentially genetically identical."

Just as astutely, Little understood that to be economically viable, you needed an organism that reproduces prolifically, has a short life span, and requires little space. After his blink-and-you'll-miss-it career as a university president (three years at the University of Maine, four at Michigan), Little retreated from academia, founding the Jackson Laboratory (JAX) in Bar Harbor, Maine, to focus on turning his creations into one of the defining scientific institutions of modern biology. Black 6 quickly became—and still is—the world's most popular laboratory mouse, one of just a handful of animals used to better understand human health. The strain, with all its quirks—unlike most mice, they have a taste for the tipple, are highly sensitive to pain, and prone to fits of aggressive barbering, shearing bald patches in a rival—would be reproduced intact into perpetuity. Less noticeably, but just as monumentally, Little's original standards of care—themselves inherited from Abbie Lathrop[8]—for his tiny charges were also passed down and became the norm for laboratory rodents.

---

8 Among Lathrop's many unrecognized scientific and technological achievements is the invention of the cage water bottle. "On some of the cages, Miss Lathrop had rigged a device for giving them water. It is a bottle with a feed tube, from which a drop constantly hangs down into the cage, and a thirsty mouse has only to stand on his hind legs to quaff a cooling drink." *Springfield (MA) Sunday Republican*, October 5, 1913.

Within a few minutes of meeting Nadia Rosenthal, the Jackson Laboratory's scientific director, I am having a weird fantasy, inserting her into my teenage life so she can be my role model. Educated at Harvard Medical School and with career stops around the globe, she is accomplished and powerful, yet natural and warm. I am in awe. What impact would it have had on my young self, who spent hours flagellating herself trying to decide on a career in the humanities, my mother's preference, or the sciences, my father's? Of course, I say none of this, but I find myself hanging on her every word, admiring her agile mix of layperson's science and personal anecdote. Not that this dexterity is unforeseeable. From the moment JAX unexpectedly acceded to my request for interviews, the laboratory has expertly controlled our relationship. First, there was the preliminary interview with a public relations (PR) specialist and the strategic communications leader, which I—no stranger to the field—navigated with peppy vagueness. Then, there are the requests for my questions so the interview subjects can "prepare." Luckily, I've honed a seat-of-my-pants interviewing style, following where the conversation leads, so could only come up with a couple, very general ideas about what I might ask. And finally, there is the presence, during my staff interviews, of the PR person herself, although she discreetly turns off the video, so all we see of her on Zoom is a black box labeled with her name. Not even were my contacts with the US military, when I was writing my first book, so tightly managed.

Rosenthal, who is an expert in targeted mutagenesis, microinjecting genetic material into one-celled mouse embryos using CRISPR, begins by impressing on me the size and scope of the laboratory: the Bar Harbor campus houses two million mice. They have more than twelve thousand mouse strains. There are three other campuses: a new high-volume production vivarium in nearby Ellsworth, Maine; another in Sacramento, California; a personalized medicine facility in Farmington, Connecticut; and an outpost in Beijing, China, a joint venture with a local biotech company. But, Rosenthal emphasizes, they are not just providers of laboratory animals, they are a serious research institute, with over sixty principal investigators, each heading up their own lab on topics as diverse as tissue growth, breast cancer, blood formation, the inner ear, and asthma. Their mice are purebreds, Rosenthal explains, with "pedigrees . . . that go back generation after generation." In short, JAX is the progenitor for all things lab mouse, from the very concept of doing research on genetically identical subjects and their patented production model[9] (US patents 7,592,501 and 8,110,721) to the twelve-story-high racks of filtered-air, autoclave-steam-cleaned food and bedding-filled box cages. "Aside from the fact that our mice are very well characterized, they're also incredibly well taken care of," Rosenthal says. "We have animal-welfare standards that really set the gold standard for animal research around the world, because we've been in this business for ninety years." I'm glad she brought this up, so I don't have to, but I don't follow up. Yet.

First I want to find out how JAX decides what to research, an activity on which it spent $462 million in 2020. "The impetus for one or another [new] model might come from anywhere—from one's own research, pointing [in] a direction in which you really feel you must go because it's been unexplored," Rosenthal explains. JAX doesn't shy away from the big questions, which often involve teams across the laboratory and outside it.

---

9 The patented JAX breeding method to prevent genetic drift in their mouse strains, already inbred through at least twenty generations of parent-offspring or brother-and-sister matings, is to refresh a naturally breeding colony from two "twin" founders every fifth generation with frozen embryos that are siblings of the original founders. This involves a short surgery to implant the embryos in a female who has been prepped for fertilization by having sex with a castrated male. Two offspring, a robust male and female, are chosen from this litter and placed in a box cage, where they will live a life of ease—no work, no danger, food and drink, and ample sex. Females will have their miniscule vaginas regularly examined with a toothpick or "blunt metal probe" for "copulatory plugs," a cream-colored mass of mouse ejaculate. Her pregnancy can be confirmed eleven days after this has been discovered, and, if successful, will result in a litter of between two and twelve, who will also enjoy a carefree existence of making merry and whoopie. Repeat five times.

"We have larger projects that involve multiple groups who are thinking in more detail about, for instance, what if we put a particular mutation that we know shows up in a human, and that predisposes them to let's say, type 2 diabetes, which is one of the big foci that we're now working on. Do we want to put that mutation on a background that is maybe, maybe relevant to humans? Or maybe not? And the answer is, since we don't know why we are choosing [it], we should put that mutation onto a number of different backgrounds so that we can understand better what the genetics is telling us about whether that mutation is really the driver. . . . I'm just using that because I know you're interested in metabolic disease. But mice are very active. Mice are not couch potatoes. They don't sit around. Unlike, you know, people. . . . I mean, you can just ask the question, how many kilometers does a mouse run on a wheel all night long? Because that's their daytime, and they love running on wheels." I ask her to hold the thought so we can finish our conversation, but I feel oddly guilty. At the outset of all my interviews, I tell my subjects that I don't practice gotcha journalism and that, if my editor lets me, I quote them fully, not just a sentence or phrase pulled out of context. But this? It's as if I'd left a trap lying around in a dusty corner of our conversation and she wandered in of her own accord. Then I ask her why she thinks mice like to run.

"Runner's high," she jokes. "You know, there are days when you start and it feels like you're dragging around a deadweight? But I think mice don't have that situation. They're not sedentary, they don't sit and talk to each other over Zoom. They are enormously active." Rosenthal, as you might expect from someone who's spent her career working with mice, has a deep understanding and abiding affection for her tiny charges. They are intensely social, she tells me, constantly interacting with one another, and very inquisitive. Because they are nocturnal, their two most powerful senses are tact and hearing. "They communicate in ultrasonic frequencies. You can record it, and you can dissect it, and it's clear that they are literally communicating. It's not just, you know, 'Oh, eagle, eagle overhead!' It's much more complex than that. And so, I think that they spend a lot of time wandering around and talking to each other." Then she returns to the theme of the wheel. "All mice, at some point or another, if you give them a wheel, will run on it."

Her theory about the origins of this proclivity is that their foraging campaigns are fraught with danger. The mouse's small size makes it a tempting morsel for a host of predators—hawks, eagles, snakes, dogs, cats, skunks, and even, from time to time, raccoons and squirrels. Which is why, Rosenthal explains, "The mouse has to be very clever about how it gets from A to B. And the best way to do that is to run like hell. I mean, it's like being in a war zone, right? You just do not saunter across a field where there are enemies in the bushes. You run like hell, and that's why war movies look like everyone's running all the time. It's the same thing for mice; they're in a constant war to stay alive."

What does that mean for their metabolisms? I wonder. "All that running takes a lot of energy, it's true, which keeps mice really light. I mean, they're only thirty-five grams. And that's not very much. They can literally subsist on half a peanut a day." Yes, I say, I've read some studies on how the caloric requirement for the amount of activity a mouse does is actually very low. "And the thing that's different about a mouse is that its lifestyle depends upon its running." I ask her how laboratories accommodate this need. "I think not well enough, not well enough." I ask her if JAX provides mice with running wheels. "Obviously, we can give them the equivalent of one of those PetCo hamster enclosures, which we have actually done. It's really interesting what happens. But we can't afford to do that if we've got two million mice to take care of." And, I think, but don't say, because JAX, the "gold standard" for mice, does not, no one else does either.

My final question: "So in terms of experiments that are conducted on animals that don't have these types of enrichment, particularly, you know, the ability to move, the ability to socialize, the ability to gnaw, how does that affect the science?"

"I mean, that's a profound question. By definition, the answer is yes, it does affect the science. The concept to date has been . . . if you have the same environment in every cage, anything that differs from one cage to another, must be associated with some variable that you're trying to measure," she says. "And this is kind of the essence of reductionist science, right? You take one variable at a time, so you can understand how that variable affects the outcome. But I think in the end, we need to understand that changing one variable at a time is probably not going to get us very far, very fast."

For that reason, JAX is revamping its model for the twenty-first century to include a product line that highlights population diversity, Mark Wanner, the director of research communications, explains to me another day while giving me a Zoom tour of the Bar Harbor, Maine, headquarters. Wanner brings me out onto a deck overlooking the park—the view of the hilly islands and bay is stunning. "There's a [cell phone] tower up here so we should be okay—although my rule is, the shoulds don't always pan out! I'm going to zoom out a little bit more again. That's Cadillac Mountain in Acadia National Park. We're right next to it—there's a park loop road that goes right there." The proximity is not accidental; George B. Dorr, a wealthy early preservationist, donated land and resources to both. "And I'm going to talk a little bit more about the mouse diversity, the genetic diversity. That's a huge direction that we're going in. Biotech—and biopharma—is a little behind us, and we're trying to get them to adopt that. But essentially, it's trying to move mouse-based research into more of a human situation where you fit in with humans, right? If you test something, it works in me. What does that say about how it's going to work in you? Not much. Our genetics are so different. And there's so many variables that you can't assume it works for everybody. But they test them in mice that are genetically almost identical. So it would be like testing a drug in me, and in me, and in me, and saying, hey, it works. And so we've developed some tools for that, which I'll discuss later."

Wanner shows me the East Research Building. There are wet and dry laboratories, which we peek at through doorways, and a long hallway. He points out Dorr Mountain and tells me that a lot of their animal care workers have to live off-island. "I'm happy to say that my wife and I own a house here, but it's just gotten ridiculous, like a lot of places during the pandemic, and you can't afford to come to the island anymore, which is too bad." He tells me that the new vivarium they are opening in Ellsworth, price tag $200 million dollars, twenty miles away will help alleviate housing pressures for the 1,600 staffers who work here. There, they will produce "the high volume ones—it's only like twenty strains. Most of them [the other ones] lose us money, and, basically, we're supported by the NIH [National Institutes of Health] to provide them for disease researchers. But most of them are high maintenance. We don't keep them on the shelf because we want to be as efficient as possible and not have mice that aren't going to be actually used. So we have minus 180 degree storage tanks full of embryos ready to revive most of our strains." He waves at an unassuming, three-story structure made of brick, concrete, and tempered glass and tells me it's the Isolation and Importation Building, where donated mice are examined and quarantined; the full basement is where they keep the medical-grade freezers with frozen embryos.

"And then we have the diversity outbred population, which is, again, you start with these eight founder strains, and you outbreed them," Wanner says, back on the topic for which I am fairly certain some talking points got circulated before my interviews. But to me it suggests that the laboratory is worried about the future of its business model. If scientists begin to reject the genetic twin model of research, then selling small populations of intentionally different mice, birth-to-death data collection and analysis using machine learning, and researching and providing personalized medicine as they are doing at their Farmington, Connecticut, campus may be just the strategy that helps JAX dominate the field past its century mark, 2029. "It's not an inbred [strain], you don't have consistency," Wanner continues. "So you have to have the tech to support it, seeing what's going on with the genomes across these populations. But you can have a population as small as two hundred of these outbred mice, and you get genetic diversity, that it's not exact, but it mimics the human population." Morbid as ever, I can't resist asking what would happen if an earthquake, hurricane, or another fire (the nonprofit was walloped by one in 1947) somehow loosed their internees into the nearby white pines and wild blueberry bushes. Wanner chortles. "I think the local—we have foxes, we have coyotes, we have tons of owls and hawks—predator population would be quite happy." But then, like a boomerang, he's back to population diversity. "It makes it much more powerful, much easier, again, to parse out within the genome why certain things are different between different strains. . . . It's expensive, you know, you have to have a lot of mice. So, and a lot more data collection, a lot more data collection."

I think back to the very first thing I noticed on the Zoom tour: the ceiling, which was lined with tubular structures. It seemed odd that an organization with the resources of JAX would have exposed plumbing. I interrupted Wanner, who was explaining that we were moving from the oldest to the newest laboratory building. "I'm sorry. I just had a question. Are those normal pipes above in the ceiling there? Or is there anything special that's being piped in?"

"Data cables," he says. "We actually had to open up some fiber-optic fiber to get a pipeline, so we could send and receive sufficient bandwidth. . . . We're talking petabytes. You've got ten thousand full genomes, and you need to match it up with RNA-seq [sequencing] data. The amount of data in biomedical research right now—it's just insane. It's so much. And so it's always like, you know, it's the treadmill that keeps going faster. You're always running really hard and not getting ahead."

I really want to like JAX. The laboratory is so well-organized and so well-run. Their staff is intelligent, friendly, articulate, and committed. They obviously care a lot about the welfare of their animals. They believe they are doing good in the world! But. I mean, I'm not a vegetarian. I enjoy a broiled ribeye, prosciutto, and pan-roasted chicken, even though I know that the meat I eat is produced by a system in which cattle, pigs, and chickens live wretched lives. Similarly, I know that many laboratory animals have suffered and died for medical research. But I received the polio vaccine as a child and one for yellow fever when I was traveling in lowland areas of Latin America. Like most Americans, I use dozens of personal care products every day—shampoos, lotions, soaps, and makeup, some of which were undoubtedly tested on mice or other creatures. But every time I plunge into the nitty-gritty of what they do, I am pulled up short.

I read the JAX website, client materials, published papers, and even talk with one of their mouse technicians, and the word *monstrous* pops into my head. JAX's surgeons not only implant frozen embryos into estrus-induced females all day, they offer a plethora of murine medical procedures to harried researchers. Mice can be delivered "pre-conditioned," "study-ready" with catheters already inserted ($117.49–$225.00)—similar to those chemotherapy patients use, but much smaller; cannulas for taking blood samples can be implanted in their brains ($283.28); or parts of their livers removed ($152.56). For customers who really want to get into the weeds and start their own colonies, the laboratory shares helpful hints. Don't be alarmed if your mouslings are born with tiny heads—the classic B6 model is prone to anencephaly. Some mutant strains, such as AKR/J (000648), C3H/HeJ, NOD/ShiLtJ (001976), and the transgenic B6CBA-Tg(HDexon1)62Gpb/1J (002810) may only produce a couple of litters before the mother succumbs to her genetic defect, be it leukemia, ovarian cysts and tumors, uncontrollable tremors and seizures, or diabetes. And, by the way, you should keep an eye on those obese-type breeders. They "are so heavy that they cannot lift themselves up to where food hoppers are normally placed. If they do manage to hoist themselves up that high, they sometimes fall over on their backs and cannot right themselves." (Their greasy appearance comes from rubbing up against their high-fat food.) Want to get a number of females to produce same-age pups? "House the females together as densely as permitted by your institution's Animal Care and Use Committee (ACUC) and induce simultaneous estrus by exposing them all to male urine." Most telling of all is the following caution about the descendants of natural mice: "Most wild-derived inbred mice are hyperactive and require special handling." I guess this means they want to run?

∞

Strangely, until recently, no one knew the answer to that question. On the occasions that a laboratory animal had access to a running wheel and hopped on to give it a spin, scientists attributed it to a need to relieve stress, frustration, and boredom related to their captivity. So, almost a decade ago, the Dutch researcher Johanna Meijer, a specialist in the study of time-related phenomena in biology, decided that she would devise a test to see if wild rodents were as interested in running as their caged counterparts. In a Zoom from her home, she gestures toward a green-filled picture window behind her. "So I have a very deep garden, you can see it here. In the very back of my garden is a wood. And I had a running wheel installed there." She also located a movement-activated infrared camera. And then she waited. At the beginning, although mice consumed the food placed nearby, nothing happened. "And then, yeah—surprise!—at some point, we suddenly saw that an animal [had come] in the middle of the night and was running on the wheel. And we were so tremendously happy. It's so weird that you can be so happy. I mean this happens all the time in the lab, but then you see it in the backyard. And it's oh, it's really happening! So the animals started to run on the wheel." Meijer and her colleagues continued recording the mice in her garden exercise station for a year and a half, then set up a second location in the dunes, in "a wild place where you can do experiments. I had electricity from all the German bunkers that were built here at the border of the sea—they were useful after all, bad joke." The same thing happened. At first nothing. Then, after a period of acclimatization, the mice and other animals visited regularly to run on the wheel—even when no treats were offered. "What we showed in this way is that [even] if animals are not in captivity, they voluntarily run in a wheel." Although her wild mice didn't spend as long on the wheel as mice in cages—who run an average of eight kilometers a day, when all their other activity is taken into account, it would be about the same, Meijer says.

"A natural amount of [physical] activity is so intertwined with the metabolic state—this is not something trivial," the scientist emphasizes. "And in fact, in conditions without running wheels, animals are kept in a kind of sedentary lifestyle. Organisms are made or have developed to be active. Being active is then interwoven with the whole physiology of their body. And if you change that level of activity, we know now that that [causes] dramatic changes—even for mood, but of course, definitely, in the first place, for metabolism, but also for sleep quality and for alert-ness and for the chances for disease. So, if you do recordings of [collect data about] animals, then it's very important and also easy, actually, to give them the possibility to have voluntary activity. And I stress [that] it is voluntary activity." Forced activity, Meijer says, not only upsets the animals, it activates different areas of the brain. She says that an ideal laboratory enclosure offers a mouse the opportunity to be active when and for how long it wants, as well as accommodates its intense need for social interaction. Meijer has designed her own cages, which consist of a central chamber for communal activities surrounded by running wheels, one for each occupant, with an entrance that only admits that particular mouse so that the time, duration, and mileage of its sessions can be tracked. "That's important if you want to relate particular physiological parameters to their health and to the amount of activity from each individual mouse—how much it has run."

Before we end our conversation, Meijer makes sure to clarify to me her stance on the use of animals in the laboratory. "I'm not against animal experiments, I mean, without animal experiments, we wouldn't have had a vaccination for COVID. Without the animal experiments that I did, I would not be able to protect biodiversity, the way I'm doing now, just by seeing how important dim light at night is. And also, a living creature and animal is really much more than a sum of cells and genes. So what I find problematic is, at the moment, the whole tendency to—because this leads to grant money—to say we can do without animal experiments, we rebuilt this data on a chip, and we have lines of cells, as if you can pretend to understand life from such a reductionistic perspective. . . . So I'm saying this to you, because it's sometimes, I find it's an easy trap, so to speak, for outsiders to, to think that it's possible to understand life and to treat diseases by just studying some cells. We can't. . . . What is important is to do the whole thing in the most humane way possible so that quality of life is very well protected."

I ask her what she's working on now and if it's related to physical activity. As part of a consortium of Dutch universities, she is investigating several issues related to the biological clock: how it affects or is affected by shift work, school hours, and light conditions in nursing homes and assisted-living facilities; how circadian rhythms relate to disease and mental health; and how artificial lighting is affecting biodiversity and the natural environment. "We have learned for the animals that if you have a very weak amount of light at night, very low level light intensity during the night, that you just already disrupted nocturnal animals to a pretty large extent, very much at the expense of their health. And now we are doing this in nature—the Netherlands is the most light-polluted country in the world."

"That's very interesting," I say. "And it makes a lot of sense. My middle daughter, who's eighteen, got terribly depressed last year. And because of the pandemic, you know, we are all studying at home. And she had blocked off her windows with blankets and she was not going outside. And I was very much worried about that aspect of it."

"Well, I noticed the situation from a personal perspective, so I feel very bad for you. But this is really what it does. And the thing is that children, especially during the pandemic—maybe you should stop recording this. But this is not talking from a purely scientific point of view anymore. But this is what I noticed . . . everybody gets up later and later and goes to bed later, because you don't have to go to school. And then people think that is good, because you live according to your clock. But you do not live according to your clock, because your clock is, humans are made to be active in the day. By the evening light [with the artificial light at night], we postpone our clock, and then we get up later the next day. . . . And what we now do and what all the children are doing is they make very short days, because they get up late. But the sun goes down at the same time. So they make days of maybe five or six hours. And this is what happens in the Scandinavian countries, from which we know there is so much depression in winter because the days are so short."

∽

It was hard to believe we'd successfully rid ourselves of our rat interlopers. The experience marked us—and the house, where, if you pull the stove and dishwasher from the kitchen wall, you will find a constellation of tennis-ball-sized holes. I found myself increasingly grateful for Rafi's tunnel-vision approach to problem solving and his general imperturbability at anything less urgent than a life-threatening illness or imprisonment (and even then, he's the first with the irreverent jokes and the audacious plans). For a couple months afterward, the girls, chastised, scrupulously washed their dishes, stored food in its place, and avoided off-hour snacking. The cat, as if she were smelling ghost rodents, occasionally leapt off the loveseat in my office, pressing her nose avidly along the baseboard and into the utility closet, then emerged a few moments later, her whiskers hung with dust bunnies, to finish her nap. Outside, the pandemic ebbed and flowed. During the summer it eased enough that we foolishly held a garden party where Rafi and our friend Paco had a heated political argument, sputtering in each other's faces, much to the horror of our COVID-19–traumatized children, and scheduled a visit from my cousin and her son from Oregon, then, as our state ratcheted up its quarantine for visitors, canceled it at the last minute. Gabi attended an online summer program on medicine; Mariela, on the other hand, after the abrupt cancellation of all her spring after-school activities, hadn't been able to enroll in a single program. (I griped about the competition for enrichment activities now that everyone was living our frugal, home-based lifestyle.) The girls socialized outdoors, always masked, and Gabi even made a couple visits to her boyfriend's closed-in porch after six months of constant FaceTiming. Life wasn't normal, but it felt summery, optimistic. Maybe we were turning the corner?

School started, which this year meant the girls powering up their laptops and joining their teachers and peers via Zoom. The days got shorter and colder. COVID-19 cases went up and up. As she has done every fall since she was four, Gabi played soccer, but this time in a mask and in a practice pod to avoid close contact with other players. When the season ended, there was no banquet—besides, Gabi had stopped hanging out with her teammates and had been turned off by her coach when she penalized athletes who were late to practice because they had to take the bus instead of being dropped off by parents. Mariela continued with her long bike rides and saw her friends on ambling, masked jaunts through the city. Halloween was canceled, although we laid individually wrapped candies on the edge of our porch steps in case a few younger trick-or-treaters came by. For Thanksgiving, the four of us prepared the meal we wanted—tostones, empanadas, *yuca frita*, and seafood paella. We briefly connected with far-flung family by Zoom, tantalizing them with our nontraditional feast. The holiday felt relaxed, not like the days of preparation, hours-long event, and inevitable overeating in normal years. Still. In the short, gray days and long, black nights hung a sense of grief—so many sick, so many dead—and fear. Gabi, who for months had badgered me at the end of every pandemic-related conversation, "Yes, but how long do you think this will last?"—disbelieving that I didn't know the answer, stopped asking. She also started spending even longer in the bathroom than normal—which, as a healthy, young woman, was already upward of a half hour. Sometimes I thought I heard sniffling.

One day I knocked. "Gabi, are you all right?" A mumble. "Can I come in?" She was standing in front of the mirror, parting her hair and peering forward. Her face was tearstained. "What's going on?"

"Mami, my hair is falling out. Look!" She ran her fingers through a patch, tightened them and pulled. Several strands came with it.

"My hair falls out all the time," I said, unhelpfully. "After I finish brushing, there's always a big ball."

"No, I mean really," she said, and proceeded to tell me the backstory: last July, she had gone to the high school health clinic and gotten a birth-control prescription. I was momentarily hurt. I am open about sex and pragmatic. With Esme, I'd arranged for her to get contraceptives when she decided she was ready to be intimate with her first boyfriend. But Gabi, who is like me outside and in, did not confide her thoughts, nor asked for my help. Fiercely—pigheadedly at times—independent, she had arranged for her own reproductive health care and adhered carefully to the medication's schedule. "It's sometimes a side effect of the hormones."

Grateful to be invited into her life now, if not before, I helped her contact her pediatrician, who arranged for a different brand of pill, one with less progestin, and we drove to the drug store to pick it up. Gabi had proudly gotten her license that spring—because of the pandemic, Rafi had taken her to a town an hour away—and usually took every opportunity to show off her skills. But today she slumped into the passenger seat. I drove even more carefully than usual, glancing at her from time to time. Her face was closed; her eyes downcast. What was she thinking about?

As always, my life was too busy. Since the beginning of the pandemic, Rafi and I had been working day and night in our public health business. This period was starting to rank up there with running a newspaper as one of the most intense professional experiences of my life. It felt good, though, I mused, like being a nurse during World War II. We were in the middle of the action, helping people, maybe even, if indirectly, saving lives. The girls continued with their remote learning and their flipped schedules. After several months of conscientiously cleaning every last scrap and smear from the kitchen at the end of their nightly food-preparation jams, they'd gotten lax. Now, when I got up, not only did I face a counter strewn with half-eaten food and a sink full of dirty dishes, I did it enraged, thinking that it was only a matter of time before the rats returned. Gabriela was busy—school, a couple shifts a week at the supermarket, and applying to colleges. Barred from getting together with extended family, I made a point of scheduling—and documenting with my camera—all our traditional holiday activities: the felt advent calendar where I tuck tiny gifts, notes, or treats in each pocket; the trip to the family-owned garden center to buy a tree (by the time we got there, the only specimen left was a scrawny pine; the rest had been picked over by the newly home-based hordes); mounting the tree and decorating it with our three generations of ornaments, from the 1940s–era angel with an electric bulb halo to the gold-sprayed macaroni wreath my sister made as a toddler (she converted to Judaism, so I inherited the family collection) and the gray porcelain cat I bought the year before Smokey died; the Christmas-light tour, driven by Gabi, in which we wove through several neighborhoods of tightly packed triple-deckers and single-family homes where the displays are obviously a good-natured annual competition; making cookies; setting out the stockings, writing a letter to Santa, and reading—Gabi did the honors—"'Twas the Night Before Christmas." I inserted letters into the stockings of all our missing family members, then sent them photos of both. On New Year's Eve, Gabriela and I reviewed her applications—of course, finding several responses and essays that had not been done—until it was time to watch the socially distant countdown in Times Square. We got through the holidays okay, I thought.

The girls spent a lot of time in their rooms. Where else could they go? Gabi had turned hers into a dark cave, tacking fleece blankets over the airy curtains, often sitting in her bed with only a dim salt lamp and the light of the laptop or phone. "Your plant is going to die!" I scolded her. In a flurry of decorating—along with a TV and an aromatherapy vaporizer, she had purchased a large palm plant, on sale from work for seven dollars, down from fifteen. "It needs light. Open the curtains every day and put it next to the window." I added a stop there to my weekly watering rounds, determined to ensure that it had its minimal needs met. Worse, Gabi, who had always been our most active child—even in the womb, she had regularly butted her head against my cervix, as if she couldn't wait to get out and tear the place apart, seemed to have reduced her daily exercise to bathroom and kitchen trips. When she was small, she was a whirlwind, which, combined with her fearlessness, resulted in her being anointed a "frequent flyer," a kid who regularly appeared in the ER to be stitched or slung up. Among our many nicknames for her was "Bola de Fuego," a reference not only to her short temper but her unceasing energy. How, I wondered, could she stand staying in her dark room all day? Gabi's bathroom sessions continued, and she talked to me incessantly about her hair. At first, I told her I didn't notice a difference. But after a while, I could see that her abundant, long dark curls had a nimbus of frizz—short hairs that had broken off. She also showed me the result of running her fingers through—as before, several individual strands, from follicle to tip, rested in her palm.

"I don't know what to do," she wailed. "They said the birth control could affect my hormones, and now changing over to another, and that it is normally a couple of months before you see improvement. But I don't want to keep losing my hair." We decided together that she would give it another month, then stop the contraceptives altogether if the shedding continued. Meanwhile, I suggested, why didn't she try going for a run every day? It would keep her healthy, get her some sunlight, and improve her mood. A couple early college acceptances came in—her safety schools. Then a new phenomenon entered my life: simultaneous texts, phone calls, and emails at 4:00 P.M. informing me that Gabriela Salcedo had been marked tardy to a class or absent for the day. When I asked Gabi about it, she told me her first period teacher was very strict and if she joined the Zoom a minute late, noted it in her records. Used to letting her manage her own life—she had always been my most responsible child, a burden imparted to her, as it had been to me, by being a year and a half older than a younger sibling, I accepted her explanation.

Besides, I was now too concerned about something else to give it much thought. Sometimes, when I went upstairs to use the bathroom during the day or to move the laundry from the washer to the dryer, I heard sobbing. I would come closer, and there would be Gabi, sitting on the toilet, lying on the couch, or burrowed into the covers in her bed, crying inconsolably. I hugged her, patted her forehead, and asked her what was wrong. Her hair. She was going to end up bald. I tried to reassure her—I did notice the breakage and that some hairs fell out, but, at least to me, her hair still looked as luxuriant as ever. Did she think she was stressed by the pandemic, by not being able to see her friends, by not knowing what was going to happen, and when it would be over? Did she think she was depressed? "No, no, no. It's just my hair. Everything else is fine," she insisted. The palm tree's fronds in her room turned brown from lack of sunlight. One day, when she wasn't there, I dragged it out to the landing under a small window, clipped off all its dead leaves, watered it heavily, and prayed.

Spring arrived, renewing our sense of potency. I began running in capris and a light long-sleeved jersey, relaxing right into my pace instead of bracing myself until my body generated enough heat. Mariela resumed her long walks with friends, and Rafi began poking around in the garden and strolling the neighborhood listening to philosophy podcasts. The national vaccination campaign, which in our state began in January 2021, with healthcare workers, was working its way through the higher-risk groups and COVID-19 rates had begun to drop. But everything wasn't fine with Gabi. I became accustomed to the afternoon barrage of school messages about her on all my devices. I got a call from her calculus teacher, who said she'd stopped participating in class. Always diligent about her job—refusing to cancel shifts for tests or family events, Gabi stopped going to work, and her already minimal socializing ceased. She spent even more time in her room, in the dark, or occasionally on the living room couch, wrapped in a fleece blanket, also with the lights out.

We had a new, heartrending routine: Every couple of days, Gabi would appear silently in my office and throw herself on my loveseat, weeping. I breathed deeply, saved my documents, and walked away from urgent emails and texts. "Sweetie." I sat next to her, stroking her muscular back and neck, an area of her body that always brought me back to her babyhood and our physical similarities. "Your hair?" She nodded. Then we took our first step in a draining dance, her pulling me toward her fixation and me tugging her away. "It's worse than ever, I'm going bald, I'm just going to shave my head," she said, all the while picking madly at her scalp. It was all those hormonal changes—one birth control, then another, then stopping. Maybe her hair follicles would never grow again.

Maybe she had alopecia. I took another deep breath. "I know you see hair falling out, but it doesn't seem like an abnormal amount to me, and, honestly, when I look at your hair, apart from the frizziness around the crown, I don't see any difference. Anyway, even if it was initially caused by the contraceptives, how are you so sure other things aren't affecting it now—like stress or not going outside? And even if not, it can only be good to address them, right? Do you want to go running with me tomorrow?" But I couldn't coax her from the merry-go-round of her thoughts and, after an hour or so, we would simply end, too sapped to continue. One day, I asked her to say the emotions she was feeling without saying anything about her hair.

"I feel powerless and out of control. I'm scared about the future. I'm sad. I don't have any hope. I don't want to be me." It was the end of childhood, the end of high school, and even, possibly, the end of her boyfriend, Washington, since his family planned to move to Georgia in June. One night, after waving small handfuls of black hair at me, she barricaded herself in the bathroom with Mariela. I heard the buzzing of the electric hair clipper as they stripped every long strand from Gabi's head. When she emerged, I was scared to look. But they'd left about an inch and a half and the effect was beautiful, fresh, and modern: the short curls framed her full lips, large eyes, and fierce eyebrows. The next day, I renewed my efforts to get counseling, although Gabi said she didn't need it, first from our healthcare provider—with the pandemic, there was a two-month wait for first behavioral health appointments—and then the school, which couldn't do anything unless she was actually failing her classes. I googled. I talked to my friends and colleagues, my siblings, Esme, niece, and nephew. "How can I help her?" I asked them. I feel so ineffectual, so powerless, so scared.

There was one bright spot in Gabi's life: Washington. The two spent all day FaceTiming, and sometimes, after a crying session with me, I would hear him gently guide her out of the blues, even getting her to laugh. Over the months of the pandemic, I had observed how kind and loyal a friend he was—and gained an appreciation for his mother, who was strict and protective of him, his sister, and little brother. Although initially optimistic about her short hairstyle, Gabi still felt ugly. On the few excursions she made—to a new dermatologist, for example, she wore sweats and a hoodie pulled forward low over her brow. I told her how I'd buzzed all my hair at her age and would often wear bows in my crew cut—guys seemed to find it cute. She stared at me impassively, then asked if we could help her buy an expensive wig made from human hair.

When it arrived, she modeled it for us. Long, black, and straight, it had obviously come from South Asia. I could see gray hairs shimmering under henna, and, although I tried hard to avoid it, could not help wondering about the circumstances of the woman who'd sold her tresses, imagining her, like Gabriela, with her shorn head hidden by a silk bonnet or a colored headscarf. I hoped that the money she'd earned had helped fix a problem in her life. Gabi wore the wig almost constantly. I'd ask her how her hair was doing. "Not well," she told me. Once, after she peeled it off after a long day, I caught her on the stairs maniacally scratching her scalp. I prayed that her follicles wouldn't be permanently damaged by the traction and the constant moist environment, but, although I reminded her, I did nothing, could do nothing. One day, she left the wig in the bathroom and I brought it upstairs to the attic and laid it tenderly across her desk, stroking the long hairs with their couple threads of gray into place. It wasn't how I'd envisioned it, but she was finding her way through. As I left and passed the landing, I noticed the palm tree had sprouted three tiny, new branches.

∽

Abbie Lathrop, whose mouse farm begot the Jackson Laboratory's original and perennially favorite strain, the B6, had a reputation for meticulous animal husbandry. Her families of mice lived in light-tight wooden boxes with straw bedding and were fed oats and cracker-barrel crackers. Their cages were cleaned regularly—sometimes by neighborhood children paid seven cents an hour. When Clarence Cook Little began his production facility, he followed suit, turning to two local industries, lumber and blueberries, which were assembling shook, rough-hewn slats, into square, flat boxes for shipping fruit, and modified their creations for mouse housing. "Researchers around the world started putting them in little shoebox cages that they would make themselves. That was just really based on what was convenient and easy to clean," explains Joanna Makowska, laboratory animal advisor at the Animal Welfare Institute. "And if you look at the cages today, they're essentially exactly the same. Nothing has changed except the materials," which are now synthetic polycarbonates injection-molded into individually ventilated cages, or IVCs, so that the occupants breathe only filtered air, eliminating the risk of airborne infections. Larry Carbone, the veterinary ethicist, says, "Everybody in the United States follows a certain rule book called *The Guide for the Care and Use of Laboratory Animals* [a document updated sporadically by a special committee of the National Research Council]. And it specifies cage sizes for animals. And even though it tries to take the tack of, these are just guidelines for professionals to think about, the reality is, when they say, a mother mouse and her litter should get fifty-one square inches of floor space, that means cage manufacturers build cages to meet the standards in that book." In addition to cramped quarters, Carbone ticks off a list of other defects: laboratories are kept at temperatures comfortable for human caretakers, not the mice, whose high surface area to volume ratio means they quickly become chilled. They may not be given nesting materials, which is both an important activity and a way to keep warm while sleeping. And they may be kept alone, in pairs, or in a very small group, with no opportunity to interact with the dozen or couple dozen individuals with whom wild mice normally share quarters.

Rats have it even worse. Carbone says that, although the standard rat cage is four times as big as that of mice, "It's not tall enough for inquisitive rats to really spend a lot of time up on their hind legs, looking and sniffing around. As they get bigger and bigger and bigger, a shoebox cage for two big one-pound rats is like, 'Okay, we got no room to move. So here's the choice: either we get split up, and we're back in solitary confinement, or we stay together and we can barely move. Because what's the third alternative? That somebody's going to pay the money to buy us a bigger cage, where the two of us could stay together, but have more room to explore and to sleep and to walk and to climb?' So there's very much this industry standard that a lot of people are pushing against. But it's super expensive to replace these cages. These plastic shoe box cages can cost over one hundred dollars a cage." Makowska says if they have a wheel, rats will run a kilometer a day, but this is just one of a variety of typical physical activities. "If they're out in a very large naturalistic yard-like setting and there's video of them," Carbone says, "they're jumping around, and they're exploring, and they're wrestling with each other. So they, too, are very active animals." Makowska highlights another problem for caged rats. "Really, psychologically, they're burrowing rodents, the hub of rat life is inside of a burrow, it's in a dark, smaller space. And so we deprive them of that. They're chronically stressed and anxious because of that. So that's a huge thing. My own research has looked at actual burrowing inside a lab—so giving them deep substrate where they can form tunnels."

Talking to Makowska and Carbone, I am chagrined. My initial curiosity about the conditions in which laboratory rodents live had nothing to do with their well-being—and everything to do with making the case that most, if not all, nutritional, obesity, metabolic, and cardiovascular studies are performed on tiny prisoners who don't even get ten minutes a day to lift weights in the yard. This enforced sedentarism may not only invalidate or skew results—it hides the important role physical activity has in regulating health. But as I began to talk to the laboratory animal experts, I saw that the issue was far bigger than just adding a running wheel to every cage. It wasn't even about better simulating the animals' ancestors' natural environments to improve the accuracy of experiments, although that might be a welcome outcome. It was that we view laboratory rodents as disposable and unworthy of concern. Which allows us to avoid acknowledging that we have designed for them a life of suffering.

Even before being born, the mice and rats have been scientifically manipulated, first by inbreeding—a learning module on the JAX website explains "most laboratory strains are now several hundreds of generations inbred. . . . [They] are essentially genetic clones of one another"—and then through genetic engineering to make them frail, sick, or unusually susceptible to diseases. We house them in bleak and inhospitable surroundings, stripping them of the simplest mammalian needs such as keeping clean, being able to move freely, and touching others. Finally, we methodically subject them to scientific protocols that range from the merely stressful to the frankly barbaric. Cancer-prone mice strains are allowed to develop uncomfortable tumors that are then treated with experimental medications. NOD (non-obese diabetic) mice may be overfed for weeks and then have their metabolic rates measured in specially designed chambers where the new surroundings and the separation from their cagemates causes them to lose their appetites and show other signs of distress. In testing mood-enhancing pharmaceuticals, rats are sometimes placed in water-filled tubes. Those that don't swim madly for their lives, but just bob with their heads above water, are deemed depressed. Other rodents will live with cerebral microdialysis catheters implanted in their brains to facilitate the in vivo gathering of data. (Instructions for implantation: "Shave head of animal prior to mounting in the stereotaxic instrument. To mount the animal in the ear bars of the stereotaxic apparatus, lock one of the ear bars at the ~5-mm position. Loosely grasp the head, neck, and upper body of the rat from above with one hand and with a free hand maneuver one ear bar into the auditory meatus. Move the ear up and down while gently pushing the ear bar until a popping sound is heard, indicating insertion to the tympanic membrane."[10]) At every point of contact with this army of manufactured mice and rats, we refuse to recognize and meet their basic needs as sentient beings.

I'm trying to find this worthwhile. After all, experiments on mice have led to incredible medical breakthroughs—organ transplants, glaucoma therapies, leukemia treatments, and obesity management, touts the JAX website. But what I sense is that the twentieth- and twenty-first-century domestication of *Rattus* and *mus* for use in research has unleashed powerful interests, absolutely none of which are aligned with the rodents' own. The fact that they have been deliberately excluded from oversight suggests that those who profit from exploitation of this vast mouse and rat horde know that their interference in normal reproduction patterns to create diseased and debilitated organisms and their treatment of these deliberately defective animals is abhorrent and, at least according to animal rights philosopher Lori Gruen, immoral. Makowska offers example after example of how we don't consider rodents to be on the same plane of existence as we are. "What we found is that if you have a mouse or a rat that is going through surgery, invasive abdominal surgery, they are much less likely to receive analgesia after the surgery compared to the same surgery if it was done in a bigger species that we find more charismatic—pigs or dogs or primates. . . . We also found they're a lot more likely to be used in greater numbers for the same type of studies. So if you're using a dog, you might use a sample size of six for a study. But if you're using a mouse or rat, you'll use three times as many. On top of that, we're looking at the types of studies that are done with them, mice and rats are much more likely to be used in the most invasive studies, studies

---

10 Agustin Zapata et al., "Microdialysis in Rodents," *Current Protocols in Neuroscience* (2009): unit 7.2.

that cause more pain that isn't alleviated, and more invasive surgeries." A final issue is that researchers don't consider how scared their rodent patients are, especially when they don't interact with them on other occasions. The Research Institute of Sweden, a state-owned institute that seeks innovative solutions to all sorts of scientific problems, is one of the few places around the world doing things differently. "They have a huge focus on handling, because that's really kind of the big missing piece," Makowska says. "But they do also house them in tiered cages, so cages where they get to engage in bigger social groups. They also put them in these activity boxes, where they even get to experience exploration. The caretakers get to know them individually—look at them, make sure everybody's okay. So that's a whole different approach that is more around what the animals need." I ask her if she would recommend that all laboratories do this. "Absolutely, like 100 percent."

The normal living conditions of the rodents used in research result not only in sad lives for them—it affects and distorts the science that is their reason for being. Keeping them in shoebox cages means "they can't really move," Makowska says. "So that hugely affects metabolism. There's some good papers out there showing that basically all your animals in cages or control animals are metabolically morbid. . . . So when you're testing drugs on them or whatever [you] use them for, you're testing it in the physiology of a sick animal. And that's, obviously, not representative." This flank group of naysayers has been active for over a decade. In 2010 Bronwen Martin, a veterinary endocrinologist now at the National Institute on Aging, National Institutes of Health, published a scathing editorial in the *Proceedings of the National Academy of Sciences*.

> Failure to recognize that many standard control rats and mice used in biomedical research are sedentary, obese, glucose intolerant, and on a trajectory to premature death may confound data interpretation and outcomes of human studies.

Fundamental aspects of cellular physiology, vulnerability to oxidative stress, inflammation, and associated diseases are among the many biological processes affected by dietary energy intake and exercise. Although overfed sedentary rodents may be reasonable models for the study of obesity in humans, treatments shown to be efficacious in these animal models may prove ineffective or exhibit novel side effects in active, normal-weight subjects.

Will researchers be amenable to increasing cage size, adding exercise equipment, providing additional nesting materials, and making other changes that would improve the lives and fitness of laboratory rodents? Doubtful. When the National Research Council issued the most recent edition of *Guide for the Care and Use of Laboratory Animals*, in 2011, there was an outcry. For the first time, the guide recommended a minimum enclosure size for mothers and offspring. "That will add $300,000 to my budget," protested one laboratory administrator, whose institution breeds mice. Another, whose facility housed two-thousand pairs of breeding rats, estimated that to replace their cages would cost between $500,000 and $750,000, according to an article in *Nature*. Besides, introducing changes to rodents' cages will be an all-or-nothing endeavor. "They do make little wheels that fit into these little shoe box cages," Carbone says—the flying saucer–style devices can be mounted almost horizontally. "But not many people use them. And, you know, from the quality of science perspective, you want to make sure that if you do something like that, and you're studying something like metabolism, well, you better make sure every mouse has a wheel. Because if you have some mice who do and some mice who don't? Well, then you're studying different animals in many ways. And if you think you can combine their data, you're probably making a mistake."

Accommodating rodents' innate need to move would not only upend current research, because the animal's daily activity and fitness level would become additional factors in experiments, it would threaten the validity of a century's worth of research conducted on animals who have not been allowed to achieve a basic level of health. Would we have had different outcomes from the millions of studies on cardiovascular and metabolic diseases, obesity and nutrition, and even cancer and genetic conditions, if the mice and rats in them had been able to run—or, even better, if they had been kept in appropriately large, complex, and engaging enclosures? The Jackson Laboratory and the field of genetics grew up together; they are deeply intertwined and mutually reinforcing. Our euphoria at recently having cracked the human, mouse, and other codes and delight at our power to shape them have not yet worn off. But in the long run, and for a world in which lifestyle diseases cause the majority of deaths, should we even be focusing on individual blueprints, genetic errors notwithstanding, when the science of prevention is so simple, clear, and universal?

∽

More days than I care to admit, I start my run feeling, as Rosenthal said, like a deadweight. It is not always physical. I am tired, discouraged, uncertain, scared. Those days, the miles loom unsurmountable. But I've learned a trick to get myself through. I ignore my brain's plea to stop and pull it away from its catalog of worries. I focus all my attention on making each step as good as it can be: a small thrust forward with the hips, or if I am going uphill, the buttocks; a mostly horizontal leap over the pavement; a slight bend to the knees as if I were dancing, skiing, or skating; a precisely placed impact; and then the controlled roll of my sole from back to front. One after another, one after another, one after another.

5

How Food Fights
Hijacked Our Health

Martha López Coleman has always been hefty. Growing up in Lufkin, Texas, her parents, both immigrants from Mexico, worked long hours, but they made sure to have family meals, cooked the traditional way, from scratch and with fresh ingredients. She wasn't athletic, but when she entered junior high and found they allowed eighth graders to skip phys ed. if they played a sport, she joined the track team. There, as did most of the bigger girls, López Coleman focused on shot put and discus, where weight and strength are an advantage. When she got to Lufkin High School, she expected more of the same, but the coach gave her a rude awakening: The school wouldn't train for field events until winter. If she wanted to be on the team, she'd have to do cross-country in the fall, running three to five miles daily to prepare for two-kilometer races. "It was punishment," López Coleman says. But she liked her teammates, and, although she didn't place, aimed to at least finish all her events, and, after achieving that her first season, to bring her pace below a ten-minute mile. "That felt like a really big accomplishment," she remembers. "I did actually lose quite a bit of weight by the time I was graduating as a senior, but that wasn't my main purpose—as losing weight isn't my main purpose now. I'll set a distance goal or a pace goal. I gotta be working towards something. But my weight isn't, and has never really been, what I'm working on."

Cut to her late teens. López Coleman left Lufkin for Hollins College in Roanoke, Virginia, a bustling university town in the western foothills of the Blue Ridge Mountains. For the first time, instead of scraping nutritious meals from meager resources, and eating whatever was put on the table, "It's a free-for-all. Literally, a buffet of food, and you can go back and eat as many times as you want to. So to go from poverty, where you have very limited resources, to having unlimited [options], I definitely indulged, so my weight went all the way up and then some."

The next phase of López Coleman's life, early adulthood, was a busy blur—one that didn't seem to have time to include physical activity. She graduated, married her high school sweetheart, worked full time, and went back to school, earning two master's degrees, one in library science from the University of North Carolina at Greensboro in 2007, the other in education from Averett University in 2009. If that wasn't enough, the couple began their family, welcoming their first daughter, in 2009, and then returned to Lufkin, Texas, where López Coleman worked as assistant library director for the city, then entered a library science doctoral program at Stephen F. Austin State University.

It was only when López Coleman finally returned to school full time that she actually had space in her day to exercise again. "I would work out, I would go put in four hours [at school], and, at lunch, I would run, and then I would do some more work. And then I would go home and be a mom. And that was the first time I trained up to a 5K, actually trying to get up to a full 10K." Then, in 2015, she was hired by St. Patrick School, which she'd attended as a child, to be principal, and that ended that—temporarily. In 2016, she had her second daughter. Soon afterward her dad, who didn't have health insurance, was diagnosed with colon cancer. She crumbled. "I just couldn't deal with it. My husband, who's seen me for all those years, said, 'You know what? Every time you get stressed, if you run or you work out, you feel better.' So he would push me out of the house. Go work out, go run. And since then, that is what I do. I run."

Today, López Coleman averages 750 miles a year. She runs 5Ks, 10Ks, and 25Ks. She runs trails, powering through mud. During the pandemic, she cut a little track in her backyard and ran around in circles. She is an ambassador for Trail Racing Over Texas and for Latinas Run, and she and another professor have a lunchtime student running club at Wiley College, a historically Black college, where she is director of library services. She is still heavy, carrying 250 pounds on her 5'4" frame. She feels great, and her numbers—heart rate, blood pressure, lipids, and sugars—bear this out.

Tell that to the majority of public health officials, medical researchers, and obesity writers, however, and they will say it can't be so. People like López Coleman are the casualties in a vicious war between experts, with the mainstream vehemently denying that overweight and obese individuals can be healthy. This conflict is so heated that those who break with the orthodoxy are attacked, as happened several years ago to a Centers for Disease Control and Prevention (CDC) National Center for Health Statistics epidemiologist, Katherine Flegal. In 2006 Flegal, a genial and straightforward soul who likes nothing so much as to ponder the arcane details of data collection and statistical techniques, published a paper with her department's analysis of the death rate for different body mass indices (BMI) categories from the National Health and Nutrition Examination Survey (NHANES), a biannual study of American eating habits and well-being. To everyone's astonishment, including her own, she found that mortality for overweight, defined as a BMI of 25–30, was about the same as or even lower than for normal weight, BMI 18.5–25. She also found that mortality for those in the lower obesity category—up to BMI 35—did not have an increased death rate. This was dubbed the "obesity paradox" and precipitated an onslaught of highbrow hate—or not so highbrow, as her leading detractor, Walter Willett, then-dean of the Nutrition Department at Harvard Chan School of Public Health (HSPH), described her work with the very-easy-to-understand term *complete rubbish*.

Willett then conducted what was essentially a smear campaign against Flegal, culminating with organizing a May 2005 symposium to critique her research. The aftermath: "So our article that year in *JAMA* [the *Journal of the American Medical Association*] was the most referenced article. And I didn't get any invitations to any schools of public health for four years," Flegal says. "You have to remember that I was centered in Washington, DC—lots of places within striking reach of the city. I can't take an honorarium, so I'm free to come talk to you. And nobody wanted that. Nobody wanted anything." She shakes her head. "I felt like people [were] just like, 'I don't really want to hear about this.' And that was kind of my experience. And I felt that we, you know, it's hard to put your finger on these things, they're kind of subtle, but that we were kind of disgraced."

Instead of turning her ferocious intellect into further exploring her unanticipated findings, Flegal spent the better part of the next decade defending the 2004 study, publishing close to a dozen articles explaining the methodological choices she made and addressing accusations of shoddy design and bias. In January 2013 she and a Canadian counterpart followed up with a meta-analysis of ninety-seven research projects that also found that those who are overweight have a slightly reduced mortality rate compared to normal-weight people. This, amazingly, sparked a second round of harassment from Willett, yet again including a conference at Harvard, in February 2013—"Does Being Overweight Really Reduce Mortality?"—to eviscerate her work. The HSPH website described the meeting as "a panel of health experts [assembled] to elucidate inaccuracies in a recent high-profile JAMA article" and included the names of invited speakers, with shaming parentheses after hers: "*Katherine M. Flegal, PhD (invited; not in attendance)*."

Almost a decade later, Flegal is still reeling from this high-impact collision, and although she claims her career was not damaged, since she was protected as a government scientist, she was effectively sidelined by her radioactivity in the public realm. To exonerate herself and underscore just how incredibly weird the whole thing really was, she took the unusual step of recounting what transpired in an essay titled "The Obesity Wars and the Education of a Researcher: A Personal Account," published in the July-August 2021 issue of *Progress in Cardiovascular Diseases*. In her introduction, she admits, "We were unprepared for the firestorm that followed." And ends, "These attacks were surprisingly effective. A small number of vocal critics succeeded in raising considerable doubt about our work while concealing major errors in the estimates that they preferred." As someone who was about to poke the same obesity-industrial complex bear—although from a position of infinitesimally less authority, her experience gave me pause. A lot of pause. Would I too be gunned down by a firing squad of disdainful academics?

∞

This was not the first food fight in the history of cardiovascular epidemiology. The field itself began with a split so wide you could drop an ocean in it—the Atlantic, to be exact. The drama began after World War II with a steep rise in heart attacks—from 1939 to 1953, the mortality rate from coronary artery diseases ballooned from 62 to 236 per 100,000, according to the CDC. Two scientists, Ancel Keys in the United States and Jeremy Morris in Great Britain, came up with two opposing theories as to the cause of this increase. Keys, already a dashing public figure with a penchant for bold projects—from the study of fatigue among Andean mountain climbers to exploring the impact of malnutrition by starving conscientious objectors, believed the upturn was due to dietary changes, in particular an increase in the consumption of saturated fats. Morris disagreed; a shift to sedentary occupations was the culprit. Both men embarked on large epidemiological studies—Keys of the eating habits of men in selected countries around the world, and Morris of the differing heart disease rates of bus drivers and conductors on London double-deckers. But just as his predecessors half a century later, Keys and his colleagues were not content with allowing possibly contradictory hypotheses to coexist while the scientific community sifted through the evidence and tried to find meaning in it. He actively shot down the Scottish scientist's work, penning "Physical Activity and the Diet in Populations Differing in Serum Cholesterol" in the October 1956 issue of *Journal of Clinical Investigation* refuting Morris's thesis without naming him.

Keys was by far the more skilled tactician and he quickly outmaneuvered Morris in promoting his belief that cardiovascular disease was linked to diet—but he also had a powerful silent partner. In 1954 the results of an American Cancer Society study, conducted by epidemiologist E. Cuyler Hammond and statistician Daniel Horn, tracking mortality in 187,766 white, middle-aged, male smokers and nonsmokers were released. While the primary purpose had been to trace the relationship between cigarettes and cancer, the researchers looked at deaths from any causes in the two groups—and found that smokers had coronary artery disease at twice the rate of nonsmokers. (During the same period as the increase in heart disease cited earlier, cigarette consumption had almost doubled, rising from 1,900 to 3,778 per capita.[11] The use of the quick-burning, mass-produced cylinders had been promoted by advertising, and, during World Wars I and II, inclusion in soldiers' rations.) The publication of Hammond and Horn's paper prompted the infamous marshalling of Big Tobacco's public relations minions to muddy the waters and cast doubt on the connection between lighting up and getting sick. Within

11 US Department of Agriculture, "Tobacco Situation and Outlook Report Yearbook," Washington, DC, October 2007.

two weeks, the masters of manipulation had formed the Tobacco Institute Research Council (TIRC), a sham nonprofit funded by the industry to invest in smoking-related health studies. While much of their work was cancer-focused, they also supported research that might deflect attention from tobacco's impact on cardiovascular health. Which brings us to a certain bantam-weight scientist with an epic ego who vociferously argued that the principal cause of the worldwide increase in heart attacks was overindulgence in steak, butter, and ice cream.

During this period, Keys was cobbling together funding for pilots for what would become the foundation of the now-ubiquitous Mediterranean diet, the Seven Countries Study. "He was a good PR person. And he was a good grant-writing person," comments Sarah Tracy, a historian of food and medicine and director of the Medical Humanities Program at the University of Oklahoma who is writing the definitive biography of the epidemiologist. "He was able to persuade people on how their interests met his own. He got money from the food industry, vitamin industry, money from the Public Health Service, money from the World Cardiology Federation, money from a whole variety of sources." In 1955 Keys hit upon the perfect partner. It was an organization with deep pockets that, as he did, wanted to pursue the diet theory of cardiovascular health and hoped international studies would prove that that single factor reigned over all the others. He quickly wrote up and mailed off an application for "comparative studies on samples of populations known or suspected to differ markedly in the incidence of coronary heart disease. . . . Populations of interest . . . include several areas in Italy, several racial groups in South Africa, two regions in Finland, Japanese in Kyushu, Japan, and in Hawaii as well as populations in the U.S."[12]

---

12 Ancel Keys, "Application for Research Grant," Council for Tobacco Research, New York, October 7, 1955.

September 16, 1955, letter from Ancel Keys to John Brock, a Cape Town,
South Africa physician who was helping him arrange a sabbatical for Brian
Bronte-Stewart, a pilot study team member. Bold added for emphasis.

Dear Jack,

As I told you over the phone, **I believe it will be useful if
you can see Dr. Robert C. Hockett before you leave. He is
the full-time man of the Tobacco Industry Research Committee**, 350 Fifth Ave. (Empire State Bldg.), New York, and
his telephone number is Lackawana 4-1440. Enclosed is a
copy of a letter I am sending to Dr. Hockett who, incidentally,
is an old friend from the days when he was Director of the
Sugar Research Foundation.

The Tobacco Industry Research Committee was formed
last year in response to the problem posed by the report of
Hammond and Horn on the first 20 months' experience in the
Cancer Society study on Smoking and Lung Cancer. . . . **The
death certificates indicated, that for the entire group coronary heart disease was the leading cause of death, far more
important than lung cancer, as we could have predicted. And
when the smokers were compared with the non-smokers, the
mortality rate from all causes combined was considerably
higher among the smokers and this was mainly accounted for
by a greater mortality attributed to coronary heart disease . . .**

All of this you know. **The important point is that the
tobacco industry** organized this new Research Committee,
appointed to it first class men with critical scientific minds,
and **gave them more or less carte blanche to expend a considerable sum of money on research** to get at fundamental facts
relevant to the effects of smoking, the characteristics of men
who smoke, etc. Their funds are on a year to year basis at present

but there is every expectation of continuing for some time and, in fact, they do not favor the short *ad hoc* project that currently causes so much waste of time and money in this country.

Here in my laboratory, we have just received a grant from the Committee for the analysis of our extensive data in the files on our CVD subjects and other men on whom we have information about smoking habits as well as their physical, chemical and personality characteristics. Dr. Brozek is in charge of this program . . .

As ever,

Ancel

September 19, 1955, letter from Robert C. Hockett, associate scientific director, to C. C. Little, scientific director of the Scientific Advisory Board of the Tobacco Industry Research Council. Bold added for emphasis.

Dear Pete:

I have just returned from Minneapolis where I attended the meetings of the American Chemical Society. . . . I had a good opportunity to . . . chat with both Brozek and Keys about the project which is about to get underway. **Keys had a good deal to say about the possible bearing of his foreign population studies on the question of smoking in relation to cardiovascular disease. . . . The quid-pro-quo for T.I.R.C. would be some special attention to the smoking angle in Japan and elsewhere with a strong possibility of exculpating tobacco relatively as contrasted with dietary factors in the etiology of atherosclerosis as part of a study sponsored primarily by the American Heart Association. It looks like a good gamble . . .**

Very sincerely,

Robert C. Hockett

The tobacco industry was on tenterhooks waiting for the results from their grants. Dr. Hockett, the president of the TIRC's Scientific Advisory Board (SAB), a mild-mannered Massachusetts Institute of Technology (MIT) chemist who, from 1943 to 1952, was director of the Sugar Research Foundation, "thinks they are on the verge of making some important discovery in connection with the relation between fat consumption and disease. . . . It will tend to exonerate tobacco."[13] Hill & Knowlton, the organization's public relations firm and the mastermind behind the industry's pseudoscience strategy, didn't bother waiting. They were already busily pitching TIRC-grantee story ideas to magazines and newspapers. Their first win came quickly, a November 25, 1956, *New York Times* magazine article by Leonard Engel, "Research Attacks the Coronary Plague." The science writer stated, "Smoking has . . . attracted little attention among researchers as a possible factor in coronary disease. . . . Diet has been an object of much greater interest. . . . One place where such evidence has been gathered is Minnesota's Laboratory of Physiological Hygiene."

By February 1958, Keys had completed his Seven Countries pilot studies, relying on two separate TIRC grants, numbers 116 and 104, and several renewals. (His team had just been given one more, number 211.) In return, the world-renowned physiologist publicly absolved smoking as a primary cause of heart disease. Ever the responsible grantee, Keys did his best to arrange to present or publish his findings, as expected by his client. In short order, charge-clearing articles graced the pages of the world's most important medical periodicals. In the December 1957 issue of the *American Journal of Public Health*, Keys pronounced, "Tobacco may exert some influence but, if so, it would seem to be minor and secondary. . . . When we come to the diet, however, a relatively consistent pattern emerges and the suspicion arises that here

---

13 E. S. Harlow, Memo to H. R. Hanmer, American Tobacco Company, July 19, 1956.

is a primary factor."[14] On the other side of the Atlantic, in the highly respected British medical journal *Lancet*, Keys admitted that in Finland, those who smoked the most had the highest serum-cholesterol levels. To avoid the implications of this correlation, however, he posited a mysterious, but as yet undiscovered, cause. "The kind of person who smokes . . . may simply be so constituted otherwise that he tends to have an elevated blood-cholesterol."[15] And one year later, in the *Annals of Internal Medicine*, the University of Minnesota team found that the steady increase in cholesterol levels from Japan to Hawaii to Los Angeles was "not accounted for by differences in . . . the use of . . . tobacco."[16]

All in all, a grand slam for the tobacco industry. Cigarette manufacturers took Keys's findings and ran with them, in the process helping to elevate the dietary theory of the origin of heart disease over that of sedentarism. With the supposed variation in coronary artery plaque in cigarette users with different diets in South Africa, Japan, and Finland, the tobacco industry was able to deflect attention from the indisputable fact that smokers' rate of death from heart disease was twice that of nonsmokers. Dispiritingly, Keys never disowned this position. Even after the Seven Countries study was completed in 1968, thirteen years after his initial contract with the tobacco industry, Keys dedicated a whole section to smoking habits, remarking that "cigarette smoking itself may not be a direct factor in the etiology of the disease; the tendency to smoke cigarettes may be associated with other characteristics of the

---

14 Ancel Keys and Francisco Grande, "Role of Dietary Fat in Human Nutrition, Diet and the Epidemiology of Coronary Heart Disease," *American Journal of Public Health* 47 (1957): 1520–30.

15 Martti Karvonen et al., "Cigarette Smoking, Serum-Cholesterol, Blood-Pressure, and Body Fatness Observations in Finland," *Lancet* 273, no. 7071 (1959): 494.

16 Ancel Keys et al., "Lesson from Serum Cholesterol Studies in Japan, Hawaii and Los Angeles," *Annals of Internal Medicine* 48, no. 1 (1958): 83–94.

person."[17] His deceptive logic was used for decades as evidence not only in the press, but in lawsuits and Congressional hearings, such as this 1976 Senate testimony: "There are geographic inconsistencies in the data on cigarette smoking and coronary heart disease. A statistical association between cigarette smoking and coronary heart disease does not occur in all populations or in all countries. Ancel Keys, et al (a) found no significant statistical associations between cigarette smoking and CHD in Finland, the Netherlands, Yugoslavia, Italy, Greece, and Japan."[18]

Almost seventy years later, we are still struggling with the murky cloud Keys and his colleagues cast over our understanding of cardiovascular health and its relation to how we live our lives. Even after spending months reading and rereading the Seven Countries Study results and follow-ups, the pilot studies, the tobacco industry lawsuit collection, and everything I can about Ancel Keys, I'm still troubled. He was obviously a genius, and the Laboratory of Physiological Hygiene pioneered not only international population studies but laboratory and diagnostic procedures, such as codes for interpreting electrocardiogram results that are routine today. But their downplaying of the potential role of physical activity seems to have been the result of alpha-male posturing. And, even worse, they apparently knew exactly why the tobacco industry funded their work and still did their bidding without concern for the millions of human lives their obfuscation would harm. So I contacted—and eventually spoke with three times—Keys's right-hand man, Henry Blackburn, a cardiologist who joined the University of Minnesota in the early 1950s

---

17 Ancel Keys et al., *Epidemiological Studies Related to Coronary Heart Disease: Characteristics of Men Aged 40–59 in Seven Countries* (Tampere, Finland: Hämeen Kirjapaino Oy, 1966), 304.

18 Committee on Labor and Public Welfare, Subcommittee on Health, "Cigarette Smoking and Disease: Hearings before the Subcommittee on Health," 94th Cong., 2nd sess., May 27, 1976.

and stayed there for his entire career, assuming the directorship when Keys retired in 1972 until 1996, when he himself retired. Blackburn is now ninety-six and the self-appointed historian for the whole shebang. I start off with the easy question: why did Keys focus so much on diet?

"The project was pretty grand to get sixteen areas in seven countries. If you're asking all the questions in the world, that would have been so grand, you would have been buried," Blackburn chuckles. "Working with starving people, he had seen the profound changes in characteristics that were considered hereditary and genetic by changing lifestyle, by changing diet, and that set him out on this course. It's things that we've thought are just constitutional: your blood pressure, your serum lipid levels, your body type—ectomorphic or endomorphic. All this can be changed by reducing your calories for three months. That was a very important factor. He was always interested in diet. He grew up in California, and he ate a wonderful diet of fruit and veggies as a child who was already very much put off by the American diet," Blackburn says. "He was a very active person. But he had done early studies on patients with high blood cholesterol. He found that a rice diet that they're using for hypertension was very effective in the forties in lowering cholesterol level. . . . He was always a physiologist, and we did all these measures. But you have to have a focus, you have to have a hypothesis. And that was the hypothesis that he began, the dietary hypothesis."

In another of our sessions, I bring up Morris and ask him why they had ruled out his theory that physical activity was one of the most important factors in heart health. Blackburn, who keeps up with his field, is well aware of the increasing attention to fitness for prevention and treatment of cardiovascular and metabolic disease, but says that when they did the fieldwork for Seven Countries, collecting precise data on cardiorespiratory fitness would have been impossible. In fact, at that point, when many jobs were still very physical, occupation itself—categorized by researchers as light, moderate, or heavy activity—was the best measure of fitness. The first write-up of Seven Countries states that "in many populations where there are large socio-economic differences between classes, coronary heart disease is reported to be much less common in the laboring class than in the middle and upper classes. . . . Because this contrast in susceptibility between socio-economic classes is commonly associated with obvious differences in the average level of physical activity, it is tempting to conclude a cause and effect relationship."[19] They then attribute these differences to a range of other influences: housing, medical care, temperature, alcohol consumption, and tobacco use, among others. Many of these factors are what we now call the social determinants of health and shouldn't be dismissed. But the Keys team cite them as evidence for why the different social classes couldn't be grouped together in an analysis, thus avoiding acknowledging that, on average, the working class had better profiles than professionals and executives in all the markers they were examining, including weight, skinfolds, cholesterol level, blood pressure, and electrocardiogram results. Later, Blackburn, eager to reinstall himself, tells me that he and another Laboratory of Physiological Hygiene researcher, Henry Taylor, had begun an ill-fated pilot of the impact of fitness training, in which men did supervised exercise in a gym several days a week, on cardiovascular health. They had trouble with a high injury rate, which would have spelled problems maintaining enough subjects for the planned seven-year project, but also found that it "turns out that if you change the physical activity, you also change the eating patterns, you also change the smoking pattern, you also change your alcohol intake, so there's no way to examine physical activity as a pure, single factor in the cohort study or trial. Once you change one, you change them all."

"Isn't that a good thing?" I ask. "That being physically active caused the subjects to make all these other beneficial changes in

19 Ancel Keys et al., "Epidemiological Studies Related to Coronary Heart Disease: Characteristics of Men Aged 40–59 in Seven Countries," *Acta Medica Scandinavica* 460, supplement (1967): 278.

their lives?" Blackburn nods, but reiterates that it makes it impossible to hold all other factors constant so you can study the impact of just one. He is now writing up a review of that work to publish in the *American Journal of Epidemiology* and after we talk, emails me an embargoed copy.

All the times we've spoken, I've avoided the tobacco topic. But now I want to bring it up and see what he says. I tell him I've summarized all the cohorts in the Seven Countries Study and found that only 18 percent were overweight or obese, while 80 percent were moderately to heavily physically active and 60 percent were smokers. Kind of the opposite of today, I say. "So I'm still puzzling, a little bit, on how to balance out the diet, smoking, and physical activity. Because it seems that when that data was collected, it was during a period where you would have had, as a baseline for many subjects, the salutary effect of the physical activity combined with the deleterious effect of the smoking. So, somehow, maybe they don't cancel each other out, but they add up and affect the overall cardiovascular health."

"That's a very important point," Blackburn says. "And a very important point for you to write about for the public. In cultures that are so uniform, in terms of their smoking, or their eating, or their activity, it's very difficult to study relationships within such a culture. Theoretically, we just say, if 100 percent of people smoked, and you were looking for the cause of lung cancer, you would find out it was genetics." He pauses. He still hasn't volunteered anything about the University of Minnesota's tobacco industry–funded work, so I keep going.

"One of the other things that seems curious to me, though, was that it seems that some of the findings of the original study were not in alignment with what we now know to be true about things—of course, about physical activity, but also about smoking. . . . Obviously now, smoking has been correlated with coronary heart disease and all sorts of conditions. And they even have a fairly good understanding of some of the mechanisms by which that happens. And so, I'm curious why, when I look back at your data, it doesn't reflect that at all."

"Ancel probably made some inopportune statements early," Blackburn says quietly. And that's all I'll get. But it's enough. "Smoking didn't really show up until the ten-year monograph and later, so, in these countries, smoking the way they were smoking, and not having other risk factors. For example, 70 percent of the men smoked cigarettes in Japan, and yet they had the lowest coronary disease rate. So, yeah. You're right by that there's inconsistencies, but there are reasons why. And actually, the mechanisms of tobacco are not that clear. Tobacco and in terms of atherosclerosis, not clear at all. In terms of blood clotting, maybe a little bit clearer. In terms of acute effect, [as a] precipitating mechanism for arrhythmia, it's very well understood. But we really don't understand why there is a fairly strong relationship in our culture to coronary atherosclerosis." I don't push it. But I know that in 1999, a couple years after Blackburn was deposed to give testimony for the huge state attorneys general lawsuit against the tobacco industry, first in October 1996 for Mississippi and then in March 1997 for Florida,[20] he quietly published a paper with his colleagues, "Cigarette Smoking and Mortality Risk," correcting the Seven Countries position. I think he is doing exactly the same thing now with physical activity. And as much as I like the guy, I know he is desperately trying to preserve their legacy, eager to patch the cracks in what is now a piece of mid-century vintage science. I've gotten what I wanted from him, an admission, however slight, that the University of Minnesota researchers understood the consequences of their tobacco analysis. I don't think he'll be able to say the same about me.

---

20 Deposition of Henry Webster Blackburn Jr., MD, October 17, 1996, Mississippi Tobacco Litigation and Deposition of Henry Webster Blackburn Jr., MD, January 20, 1997, *Florida v. American Tobacco Company.*

∞

When I catch up with Flegal via Zoom, I see immediately that she trusts—has always trusted—her own research. The epidemiologist is unapologetically plump, with a broad, comfortable smile. I ask her to explain why so much vitriol was directed at her. Ever the scientist, she is careful to frame her remarks as speculation, but my question obviously touches a nerve. "There's a lot of financial interests, in terms of career interests, and I think that is actually the motivation, not just with the Harvard School of Public Health, but with other people. . . . The mortality article came out in 2004. And it got a lot of publicity. And, you know, [that was a time when experts were saying that] obesity is going to overtake smoking as a cause of death. And so then we come out with our article, which says, this is really a much lower number, and it got a lot of media attention, a lot of coverage, really a lot of coverage. I don't think people liked that." I don't interrupt her, but I know exactly what she's talking about. I've been researching it, too: an unholy alliance between obesity experts, whose careers are founded on the idea that fatness is what ails Americans (and peddling their various cures), the medical profession, and the pharmaceutical industry. "All these people think that's a really terrible message to weigh in on. But they can't say you shouldn't have published your article because of this potential message. [So] they say something's wrong with your article [because they can't say] you should have self-censored. And I know there's a lot of self-censoring going on in all this obesity research area," Flegal continues. "You have to say all these things to show that you're on the right side, or the wrong side, or any side. We just say, here's our numbers. People found that very disturbing. . . . I think there was this kind of feature that was just like, who's in charge? Who controls the narrative?"

Timing is everything, and it bears remembering that in 2012, just before the publication of her meta-analysis, the American Medical

Association (AMA) had been asked by the American Association of Clinical Endocrinologists, the Endocrine Society, the American College of Cardiology, the American College of Surgeons, and the American Heart Association to declare obesity a disease. Flegal's work, which found the harms of excess weight exaggerated or nonexistent, threatened the underpinnings of this push—and the very legitimacy of diet-focused obesity work. In June 2013, after much controversy and outright opposition from many of its members, the American Medical Association did vote to call obesity a disease. Almost immediately, a joint task force consisting of the American Heart Association, the American College of Cardiology, and the Obesity Society was formed to create guidelines for lifestyle interventions, surgical procedures, and pharmacological treatments for these newly sick patients, coauthored by Willett's collaborator and current HSPH Department of Nutrition chair Frank Wu. The way was now legitimized for physicians to diagnose excess adiposity as a medical issue, prescribe pills that profited the pharmaceutical industry or surgery that filled the wallets of bariatric surgeons, and for insurers, particularly government programs susceptible to insertions from lobbyists, to foot the bill. After our interview, Flegal and I exchange chapters from our works in progress on the medicalization of obesity; they are eerily similar, although she has focused more on the science and I, on the politics.

Flegal declines to interpret her findings, but others have taken a stab at doing so. The consensus opinion is that having a few extra pounds confers a buffer, especially as people age, that helps you weather illnesses. But when I look at her tables, I immediately notice that neither physical activity nor its more accurate cousin, cardiorespiratory fitness, is a variable. I wonder what the average fitness level was for each BMI category—underweight, normal weight, overweight, and obese—and if that might help explain Flegal's "obesity paradox." After hours of browsing PubMed and a few emails, I turn up just a handful of studies. The first,

"The 'Fit' but 'Fat' Concept Revisited: Population-Based Estimates using NHANES," published in 2010 by Glen Duncan, now a professor at the Elson S. Floyd College of Medicine and chair of the Department of Nutrition and Exercise Physiology at Washington State University, seems custom-made to answer my question. Using a sample of five thousand adults for which he had data from submaximal exercise tests (maximal measures cardiac output after exercising to exhaustion; submaximal, for a limited duration of time), Duncan extrapolated the results to the entire US population. His findings, when I examine them by BMI category, shock me so much that I barrage him with emails to make sure I'm understanding correctly: 67 percent of normal-weight people were considered highly fit, 50 percent of overweight, and a full 44 percent of obese individuals. Mind you, his sample only included ages 20–49, dropped out the underweight category, and the definition of high fit was at or above the sixtieth percentile for age and sex in the Aerobics Center Longitudinal Study (ACLS; more on it below). But still! His reply arrives within an hour: "Yes, within the obese BMI group, roughly 44 percent were classified as high fit."

Duncan's data paints a very different picture than the one of the lethargic couch potato that still seems to underlie many depictions of heavy people and the weight loss counseling they endure. And if his estimates are accurate, it would go a long way to explaining why people with a few extra pounds are as often healthy as slim people and why the obese are not dropping like flies as predicted. Then I find another study, "Inadequate Physical Activity and Health Care Expenditures in the United States," which examines BMI category by physical activity as a way to make the case that getting people to exercise is the cheapest intervention around. The lead author, Susan A. Carlson of the CDC's Division of Nutrition, Physical Activity, and Obesity, also used NHANES data. Carlson and her colleagues found that about half the normal-weight and overweight categories were sufficiently active, 51.1 and 47.0 percent, respectively, whereas among those who were underweight and obese, only a third were sufficiently active, at 35.9 and 36.8 percent. I'm no statistician, but it's fairly obvious that if cardiorespiratory fitness is strongly associated with day-to-day health and better long-term outcomes, that the two categories in which half of the individuals get enough exercise will do better than the two in which only a third do. These are the same BMI categories that have the lowest mortality in Flegal's NHANES study and later meta-analysis. I'm bolstered in the thesis of this book, but traumatized by Flegal's story. The only way I dare make the case against the false prophets of diet-focused health is to conjure up a crowd of physical activity experts to stand in front of me on the platform. Then all I have to do is step back and let them do the talking.

There may only be a handful of population studies showing the average level of fitness within each BMI category, but there are plenty of studies that show cardiorespiratory fitness is much more important to health and longevity than weight. One of the most recent was written by longtime size-inclusivity warrior Glen Gaesser, a Greyhound-lean (he's a marathoner) exercise physiologist at Arizona State University. In 1996 Gaesser took a sharp turn away from the establishment view of the origins of and antidote for the emerging obesity epidemic, publishing *Big, Fat Lies*, debunking the idea that weight loss leads to health and describing some ways it is actually harmful. His most recent paper, coauthored with colleague Siddhartha Angadi, reviews and synthesizes the literature on weight loss and physical activity. They conclude by recommending a "weight neutral strategy for obesity treatment"—translation: forget about dieting, and focus on getting fat people healthy through exercise. They give five excellent reasons, which I will quote so as not to get them wrong:

1. The mortality risk associated with obesity is largely attenuated or eliminated by moderate-to-high levels of cardiorespiratory fitness (CRF) or physical activity (PA).

2. Most cardiometabolic risk markers associated with obesity can be improved with exercise training independent of weight loss and by a magnitude similar to that observed with weight loss programs.

3. Weight loss, even if intentional, is not consistently associated with lower mortality risk.

4. Increases in CRF or PA are consistently associated with greater reductions in mortality risk than is intentional weight loss.

5. Weight cycling is associated with numerous adverse health outcomes including increased mortality.

Hallelujah! I immediately contact Gaesser for an interview.

The article, he tells me, is really both a culmination and vindication of *Big, Fat Lies*. "It took about a year in terms of getting everything together, and it kind of morphed into something bigger than I initially envisioned. And yeah, the overall theme was basically, you know, we've been on this diet roller coaster for decades. And despite our efforts to lose weight, and the increased prevalence of weight loss attempts over the last several decades, the obesity prevalence has tripled in the last thirty or forty years here in the United States, and worldwide as well. So it doesn't seem like a weight-centric focus to treat weight or obesity-related health conditions seems to have been all that effective. I wanted to take a look at this from the research standpoint. And so we looked at all the studies that have been published, looking at changes in physical activity or increases in physical fitness and their association with improved mortality risk and compared those with studies that have been done for intentional weight loss," he says. "The intentional weight loss literature is very spotty, very inconsistent. And compared to that, the physical activity literature and fitness literature was far more compelling, far more convincing and consistent. So therein lies the essence of our piece that it is far better to be fit than it is to be thin."

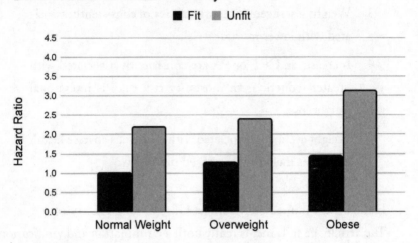

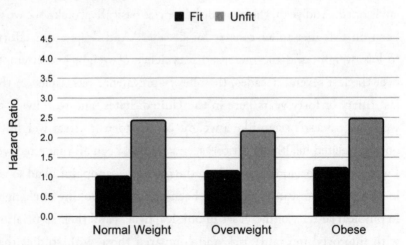

Cardiorespiratory fitness, body mass index, and mortality risk. Reprinted with permission from Glenn A. Gaesser and Siddhartha S. Angadi, "Obesity Treatment: Weight Loss versus Increasing Fitness and Physical Activity for Reducing Health Risks," *iScience* 24, no. 10 (October 2021): 102995.

I tell Gaesser about my conversation with Flegal—he interrupts, "I've known her for years"—and ask him if anything like that has ever happened to him. He appears to have emerged fairly unscathed, which I guess has to do with the combination of being male and not being the employee of a highly visible government agency. "The Harvard people just seem to have been obsessed with Katherine Flegal and her studies, because it's not just one article, you know, she's published several articles along the way on this. But I think it was basically a crusade to undermine her work. And that article ["The Obesity Wars and the Education of a Researcher: A Personal Account"] that she wrote was terrific, because it basically got behind the scenes, looked at efforts on the part of certain individuals, particularly Walter Willett, and with regards to try to undermine her credibility. And I remember after the big article she published, it created quite a stir, they had a little symposium at Harvard, to kind of set the record straight. Well, she wasn't even invited to defend her work. So it was basically like, this wasn't to air our grievances, it's basically to show that Katherine Flegal's work was just unacceptable to the scientific community, particularly those at Harvard."

I ask him the same question I asked Flegal: "Why the high level of vitriol?"

"When I'm thinking about this and talking to my students—and they asked the same thing after reading the articles: 'Why is there such resistance to this?' And I immediately say, 'Look, the weight loss industry is a huge, powerful, multibillion-dollar-per-year industry. They're not going to like this message. Because, and I quote Upton Sinclair from over a century ago, what he said is, "It's difficult to get a man to understand something when his salary depends on him not understanding it."' And I think that's just so true, that this could have financial repercussions, if everyone suddenly said, 'Hey, you know, I don't think I'm going to diet anymore. This makes sense. I'm going to just start to exercise. And I know that the fitness and physical activity will do me well, and I'm not

going to go on another diet again.' Well, that would have big repercussions financially for weight loss clinics, diet programs, you know, just
anything selling diet products, diet books. But we think it's pretty hard
to refute this evidence that we published because it shows that increasing
physical activity and fitness appear to have much more compelling effects
or associations with reduced mortality risk compared to weight loss."

Gaesser stresses that "unless you include fitness and your assessment
of health, or physical activity, you're really not getting a full picture of
a person's health. So this notion of a healthy obesity phenotype, which
is was defined, you know, a couple decades ago, this notion of a healthy
obesity phenotype came into existence. And it's largely due to the fact that
there are, there's a segment of the obese population that have relatively
low risk of cardiovascular disease. They don't have metabolic syndrome,
for example, and they are classified as metabolically healthy. But those
studies don't include fitness or activity. So it's really not looking at the
complete picture of a person's health." We chat about how that could
be done. Could there be a treadmill or stationary bicycle in the doctor's
office, maybe in the area where the medical assistant has you step on the
scale and lean back against the ruler? They could monitor you as you jog
or pedal to make sure you were okay, while the machine could collect and
analyze your exhaled breath. We agree that that sounds neither affordable
nor feasible, and Gaesser says, "But I think annual checkups should [at
least] include questions about physical activity. There are short question-
naires that have been developed that only take a few minutes asking just
a few questions about activity, how frequently do you do the following,
and it could be walking briskly, engaging in sports play, things like that."

All this is not to say extra weight, especially in the two highest
classes of obesity—there are three: the first is a BMI of 30 to under 35;
the second, a BMI of 35 to under 40; and the third, a BMI of 40 or
higher—is good for your health. If you are inactive and obese, you are
much more likely to develop metabolic syndrome, diabetes, high blood

pressure, high cholesterol, heart disease, and many cancers. This is borne out by López Coleman's experience, who noticed that when she had an extended period of inactivity, "my heart rate was a lot higher," as was her blood pressure and other vitals.

To understand the interaction between cardiorespiratory fitness and weight, I talked to Steve Farrell who, in some guise, has been working on the issue for over thirty years at the Cooper Institute in Plano, Texas. The Cooper Institute was founded by Kenneth H. Cooper, a medical doctor and air force colonel who, among other things, designed a fitness regime for astronauts to use in space, a system he dubbed "aerobics" and then wrote about for the general public, publishing the 1968 bestselling book by the same name. Instead of continuing his military career, Cooper took his earnings and founded a nonprofit dedicated to research on physical activity, a business helping public and private clients start employee fitness programs, and an on-site weight loss and exercise center. Their self-funding and single-minded focus has put them slightly out of the mainstream, and press coverage of Cooper and his brainchild tends to toggle between adulatory and mocking. But one thing is undeniable: no other place on earth has tracked, with rigorous measurements and meticulously maintained records, the physical activity, cardiorespiratory fitness—patients get a maximal treadmill stress test every time they visit, and related health variables of so many people for so long.

Since 1970, the Cooper Institute has collected information on 116,000 people, which, it says, represents over 2.2 million person-years of observation. Farrell is one of a tiny core of scientists whose job it is to find meaning in all this data, although, as he says ruefully, "Between 90 and 95 percent of Cooper clinic patients are white, and the vast majority of them have a college degree. So that's a limitation in our data that we always acknowledge in our papers."

"I'm interested in a lot of things, but one of the things I'm very interested in is the fitness-fatness relationship. And not only me, but other

Cooper Institute [personnel] have published in that area. And what we tried to do in our studies is to tease out the relative importance of cardiorespiratory fitness, versus different measures of weight status, not only BMI but also waist circumference," he tells me. Farrell, like most of the people I've spoken to for this book, exercises regularly— he walks, bikes, and does strength training, but over Zoom at least, he appeared round-faced and not particularly slim. Nonetheless, what he and his colleagues have found is that "cardiorespiratory fitness is definitely a very strong predictor of all-cause mortality, cardiovascular disease, mortality, and cancer mortality, and the same is true of obesity. But when you put the two together . . . generally speaking, those that are fit within a given adiposity category tend to have significantly lower risk of mortality than those that are unfit. Being normal weight does not necessarily put you at low risk. And being overweight doesn't necessarily place you at high risk. You have to take cardiorespiratory fitness into account." Farrell concludes by telling me that "we think it is important whenever you're talking about body weight, body size, waist circumference, BMI, however, you're going to measure body fatness, that whenever possible, when you're trying to get across that person's level of risk, you should also either have an estimate or a measurement of their fitness level. Because going by BMI by itself can be misleading, especially if a person is fit versus unfit."

"I see the difference between someone who is skinny and doesn't exercise and somebody who is obese and doesn't exercise as just a matter of time and speed," I say. "The skinny person might have a little more time before they start to have problems, but if they're not exercising, they're going to have physical problems."

"Yeah, I think that's a fair statement," Farrell says. "When we look at the degree of risk, we tend to see the lowest risk in fit, normal-weight people. We tend to see the greatest risk in unfit, obese people. And the other possible categories, let's say normal-weight unfit and obese-fit, those would be somewhere in the middle. So yeah, I think your state-ment is correct."

∽

Over the last few years, I've noticed a disturbing trend. Friends and family who previously attended dinners and parties with a lighthearted joie de vie and, once a beverage had been situated in their hands, were disposed to conversation, now arrive with a single purpose in mind: dive-bomb the buffet or table. They look better than ever: slim, glowing, and energetic. But they have been fasting for twenty-four hours and the witching hour has come: the 180 minutes a day when they are allowed to feed. As soon as they come in, their gazes dart about furiously, looking for the edibles. They nibble the hors d'oeuvres as I am plating them and before I can pass the platter to the other guests. They sometimes simply serve themselves a heaping plateful from the serving bowls and sit, alone, to devour it while the other invitees straggle in. They are practitioners of the latest diet and well-being trend, intermittent fasting, an approach to extending longevity researched and advocated by Mark P. Mattson, who for many years was chief of the Laboratory of Neurosciences at the NIH's National Institute on Aging. Among Mattson's many interests was the distorting effect of doing most of our medical research on sedentary and obese rodents, so I had spoken with him when I was researching the laboratory mice and rats chapter. But, as do most of my interviews, our conversation mean-dered. Eventually, we found ourselves talking about his work on calorie restriction, which he found protected rodents against heart attack and stroke, possibly because it reduced reactive oxygen species. Mattson, as you would imagine, is whisper thin and our Zoom conversation took place as he basked in the sun in his yard, his lawn chair inclined against the wall. As we wrapped up, I said, "So, I want to ask you a question. Can you compare endurance exercise to fasting?"

He didn't hesitate. "Exercise is much better for you than fasting, I think. And that's based on a lot of data from animal studies and human studies. And my own personal experience."

"What was that?"

"A couple years ago I tore some muscles. Initially, playing pickleball, but then mountain bike riding. . . . I didn't know it for a long time, but [they were] completely detached. . . . And so I had two surgeries. And bottom line is I haven't really been able to get—except for some walking—any aerobic exercise. And initially, I got depressed. This is actually common in people who have adopted exercise, which has an antidepressant effect. Yeah, that elevates your mood and calms you down, reduces anxiety levels. Then, if you're not able to exercise, your anxiety levels go up. . . . So anyway, at least from the standpoint of the brain, muscles, and, and even the cardiovascular system, exercise is much better [than fasting]. For example, before all this happened, my resting heart rate was in the low fifties. And my blood pressure was, like 100/60 or 110/70. And now my resting heart rate's up in the midsixties and my blood pressure. . . . Last time I had it [checked] was like 150/86. Yeah, if I had to choose one or the other, it would absolutely be exercise."

6

Treadmill-Trotting Pigs

I lean into the mirror, my glittery earrings dangling forward, and feather brown pencil into my brows. A little more than usual because it's nighttime and a party. My outfit's perfect, pretty but comfortable, a plunging net top with huge black, gray, and orange flowers; black jeans; and short boots. "Rafi, come upstairs and get ready! We have to leave in fifteen minutes!" After several entreaties, he does, muttering that he doesn't want to go. I pay him no mind. He always protests, and then, after I get a series of postmidnight texts from the girls—"Where are you guys? It's late. We're scared"—I have to drag him from his perch in front of the fire pit with the other men, leaving behind a half-drunk glass of whisky, a smoldering Dominican cigar, and the last toke of marijuana. Rafi tries on half a dozen combinations of pants, shirts, and shoes while I watch him, increasingly impatient. It's not like our friends expect punctuality. We have a running joke about predicting who will arrive the latest—one hour is common, and even up to two. Still.

When we get there, the fiesta is in full swing. Núria greets us at the door with double-cheek kisses. "¡Qué gusto verlos!" We have been friends for years, ever since, when our children were small, we formed a bilingual families group so that our children could hear Spanish being spoken outside their homes. Our monthly get-togethers quickly morphed into *botar la casa por la ventana* events,[21] overflowing with good food, wine, and music—and continued after our kids started going off to college. This party is no exception. Every room of the small house is filled with people, some with New Year's hats, black or metallic masks, and noisemakers. We weave through the crowd to the kitchen. There, on the narrow island that runs parallel to the stove, sink, and dishwasher, and surrounded by a throng, as if it, too, were a guest, presides a magnificent *jamón ibérico*. It is trussed into a *jamonero*, a special contraption for cutting paper-thin slices off the bone. The air-cured leg rests diagonally, meaty haunch on a wooden platform and black, cleft hoof waving jauntily in the air. The whole thing is encased in a thick layer of fat, amber on the outside, and one side is sliced open, exposing a pool of ruby flesh swirled with white. Bruce, Núria's husband, waves a long, narrow knife. He gestures to the forest of bottles on the counter. "What do you want? *Tinto?* White? Have some jamón!"

Our friends' holiday ham, which may or may not have entered the United States illegally in a suitcase, is a long-standing Spanish tradition. Purchased before Christmas, it is prominently displayed at all gatherings and—a measure of Latin conviviality—often finished by the start of the New Year. Spaniards trail only the Danes in per capita pork consumption, although there's an ugly side to the Iberian passion for things porcine. After the expulsion of Jews in 1492 and the forced conversion of Muslims, the consumption of pig meat, prohibited by both cultures, became a signifier for Christianity. During this period, butcher shops began hanging a ham outside like a three-dimensional religious flag. There are thousands of cured-ham producers in Spain today, the majority of which are the prosaic *serranos*, made from traditionally raised white pigs fed on cereals. The remaining 10 percent are *ibéricos*, Black Iberian pigs, a small,

---

21 *Botar la casa por la ventana* means "to throw the house through the window." It is used to describe the all-out attitude to entertainment common in Latin America and Spain.

dark, and wiry breed that probably entered the region three millennia ago with the Phoenicians, where they interbred with wild boars. They are consummate foragers, roaming the oak forests between Spain and Portugal to devour acorns. This special diet, it is claimed, imparts a distinctive flavor and healthfulness to the meat, which is richly marbled with monounsaturated fats, the same kind found in olive oil, earning the pigs the moniker *aceitunas con patas* (olives with feet). The ham—dense, rich, and aromatic—melts on my tongue. It is the opposite of American pork, the flesh of which is pasty, watery, and has a faint sickroom smell—the taste, I think, of an animal born to roam freely, that has instead lived in a cramped pen.

When Gabriela was born, in contrast to her lanky sisters, she shot out of the birth canal like a cannonball. She was also shaped like one. Picking her up the first time, I felt a ruff of flesh under her back and neck. I recognized it immediately. She had my body, which, while trim, is capped by an even layer of fat, and, when I inhale too deeply around bread or other baked goods, inflates at the behind and thighs. Gabi would grow up to be a pear. Rafi and the two other girls, by contrast, are classic apples—long, slender limbs, but with a tendency to develop paunches. Most people know that where you accumulate fat seems to be linked with its risk level: pears, padded all around with subcutaneous stores, are apparently healthier than those with protruding potbellies. This is because abdominal, or visceral, fat is "more active in producing hormones and chemical messengers that cause inflammation throughout the body," and especially affects nearby organs such as the liver and heart, explains Joann Manson, an endocrinologist and head of preventive medicine at Brigham and Women's Hospital in Boston, in a 2008 interview on National Public Radio.

Two other, less well-known types of fat deposits also hold important clues about someone's overall metabolic health: whether you have fat in between your muscles and inside your muscles. Intermuscular fat is pure bad news; it is common in those with insulin resistance, stroke and spinal cord–injury survivors, and elders with mobility issues. Intramuscular fat, on the other hand, is a mixed bag. It's present in the tissue of people with obesity and diabetes—and also that of runners and other practitioners of endurance sports, a seemingly inexplicable finding called the "athlete's paradox." A paradox is just a puzzle by another name—and who doesn't like a puzzle? I immerse myself in dozens and dozens of lipid studies of fit, unfit, lean, obese, and diabetic subjects until the pieces fall into place.

People who exercise regularly need a source of fatty acids as close as possible to their mitochondria to offer quick and ready fuel for aerobic metabolism, the kind that relies on oxygen, produces thirty-six adenosine triphosphate molecules (ATPs) of energy, and is vital for stamina. In someone who is lean and not particularly fit, these deposits don't occupy much of the cell—just 0.5 percent by volume. In endurance athletes—and obese and diabetic individuals, the droplets accept a lot more fat, but even so, they can't increase beyond about 3.5 percent of the cell by volume. Athletes deplete their droplets almost daily. As soon as they reach a steady, moderate level of exertion, their muscle mitochondria burn a combination of fatty acids, both from the droplets and the bloodstream, and glucose. The glucose, the uptake of which is mostly triggered by the exercise pathways researched by Laurie Goodyear, comes largely from outside the cell and can enter it at a rate up to fifty times greater than at rest.

But obese, sedentary people never empty these stuffed-to-the-gills reserves. No matter how much insulin is released to instruct skeletal muscle cells to take in more glucose, there's nowhere for it to go—it's like trying to top off an already full tank. Viewed through this lipid-storage lens, I start to have a radical idea. Should we even group the two diabetes together? Type 1 is an autoimmune disease, occurring when the pancreatic cells that produce insulin are attacked and destroyed; it requires a lifetime of replacement insulin injected at mealtimes.

But maybe type 2 diabetes has less to do with insulin resistance, considered its primary characteristic, and is simply—or at least, starts out as being—chronically overloaded lipid droplets. And the only way to clear them is to get moving. "The vast majority of diseases attributed to the obesity epidemic could be prevented and certainly could be treated by physical activity," says P. Darrell Neufer, Director of the Diabetes and Obesity Institute at East Carolina University. A hallmark of the *jamón ibérico* is a marbling of fat so fine that it resembles wispy clouds. During their *montanero*, the finishing stage, the swine roam their native habitat, an open plain sparsely dotted with oaks, in search of nuts. In doing so, they traverse an estimated twelve to fifteen kilometers a day. I'd be willing to bet a Cinco Jotas bone-in ham, $1,080 on Amazon, that their delectable flesh is the result of something that their cage-bound American counterparts are deprived of—not an acorn-based diet, but physical fitness, as evidenced by the Milky Way of tiny fat droplets sprayed across their muscle cells.

∽

Whenever I can, I do my errands as my daily run. I go by the bank on my neighborhood circuit with checks to deposit zipped into the back pocket of my Lycra capris. I lope the mile to the branch post office, wait in the inevitable line, and order sheets of beautifully decorated stamps, then trot through the city streets clutching my glassine envelope. I sprint to Whole Foods, a cloth grocery bag clutched under my arm, then stagger the half mile back home with it brimming with four packs of 365 Morning Buzz coffee, a half gallon of milk, and two baguettes. And when I have medical appointments, I jog to one of the two network health centers within a two-mile radius, most recently for my annual physical. After a minute or two in the waiting room, the medical assistant called me in, weighed me, measured me, and took my heart rate, blood pressure, and blood oxygen levels. "Sorry I'm sweaty," I told her. "I've just been running." She handed me a crimson johnny and left the room, telling me my doctor would be with me shortly. When she came in, my physician asked if there was anything I wanted to talk about. "No, nothing. Everything's good," I told her. "Although I'm worried about my middle daughter's mental health. She's really depressed, and we can't get her an appointment—the pandemic and all." She recommended some self-care apps and handed me a radiology slip, saying that it was time to do some bloodwork, since my last tests had been five years ago.

I got the results on their online platform the next day. My cholesterol, at a little over 200 mg/dL, had been flagged as high. My blood sugar reading, at 117 mg/dL, was borderline. Why was I, who runs four miles a day, setting off alarms? I'd apologized to the medical assistant for my clammy arm, but after she left the examination room, I availed myself of the soap dispenser, sink, and paper towels to tidy up before putting on the johnny. So I didn't bother to mention to my doctor that I'd run there. Big mistake. Exercise radically transforms what happens in our bodies at the cellular level—in the moment, afterward, and, if done regularly, long term. During my nine-minute miles on the way there, my blood circulated three to four times faster than at rest and my metabolism increased tenfold (at maximum exertion, this can be a hundredfold). Regular aerobic activity makes the heart and arteries bigger, so more blood is pumped in a single heartbeat. It also increases the blood volume itself and the density of capillaries into which it can flow. The brisk circulation—think of a fast-flowing river compared to a sluggish one—and the molecular signals that keep it moving help to keep my endothelium, the lining of my blood vessels, smooth and flexible, contributing to my overall health. But while my cardiovascular system is in high gear while I'm running, it quickly recovers. So in the few minutes I sat in the waiting room, my blood pressure and heart rate had dropped to normal.

At the metabolic level, however, my body was still in overdrive. At my relatively plodding pace, much of the energy generated by my mitochondria—the quantity of which can be doubled by endurance training—comes from combusting free fatty acids (rather than the fast-burning glucose used for sprinting). Since I'd only eaten a handful of pecans and raisins all day and it was then close to 2:00 P.M., my body would have drawn fuel from the lipid stores inside my muscles and adipose tissue. Once I stopped running, these fats remained at elevated levels, accounting for the higher reading. But the low ratio of total to HDL cholesterol showed that, in the moment, my body was actually ferrying the extra fats to the liver to be removed. "Aerobic exercise training also increases the plasma concentration of large HDL particles . . . [which] removes deposits from arteries," explain Manson and Shari Bassuk, also a researcher at Brigham and Women's Hospital, in a 2005 paper on how physical activity reduces your risk of heart disease and diabetes by 30–50 percent.[22] In addition, regularly pulling fat out of storage for use—which happens every time I run—reduces its toxic qualities, even if you have very high levels, resulting in less inflammation, better-functioning mitochondria, and better insulin sensitivity. There is a similar reason why my blood sugar was slightly high. Digestion of the raisins in my prerun snack, plus my body's increased release of glucose to help fuel my activity, had temporarily elevated them. The exercise-induced fuel-burning changes don't stop after I stop moving. My metabolic rate and ability to process glucose remain higher for the next twenty-four hours—basically, until I hit the pavement again the next day. Over time, this has made my heart and skeletal muscles even more efficient at burning fatty acids and more sensitive to insulin. (Among other heart-healthy impacts, exercise increases the production of sirtuins, which regulate metabolism and extend life spans—they are what ascetics are trying to stimulate with intermittent fasting and hedonists, with red wine.) The most radical

---

22 Shari S. Bassuk and JoAnn E. Manson, "Epidemiological Evidence for the Role of Physical Activity in Reducing Risk of Type 2 Diabetes and Cardiovascular Disease," *Journal of Applied Physiology* 99, no. 3 (2005): 1193–1204.

thing affecting a sedentary person's serum lipid and glucose levels, on the other hand, is what, when, and how much they eat. But a healthy, active person's metabolism is in an almost constant state of flux, and, depending on the moment, their blood work will result in wildly different readings. And if you aren't putting your body through its metabolic paces every day, you won't be healthy. It's that simple.

※

I used to jokingly call my mother the million-dollar mom. That was probably a gross understatement. Over the course of her lifetime of illnesses and conditions, an incalculable amount of money, first from insurance and then from Medicare, had gone into keeping her alive. There were operations and procedures—to remove tumors, to clean bone channels, to fuse disks, to insert replacement joints. There was an endless procession of appointments with specialists—endocrinologists, cardiologists, neurologists, ophthalmologists, radiologists, rheumatologists, geriatricians, and surgeons of all stripes—in addition to regular, preventive medicine. There were visits from nurses and therapists. And then there were the drugs, probably over twenty, including prescriptions, over-the-counter remedies, and vitamins. She had been told in her early fifties, when she had a stroke, that she would probably not live long. So we were all surprised and delighted when she made it to her seventies—at which point, her decades of heart disease finally caught up with her.

It wasn't like she hadn't taken care of herself at all. But like many people, she'd focused almost exclusively on diet. She was a steadfast adherent of flavorless 1970s diet foods—cottage cheese, dry toast, and low-fat everything; scooped out her portions with half-cup measures; and always ordered Diet Cokes. But the other side of the equation? There was the briefest foray into running—with a friend, several times around the block, both wearing sandals. Then nothing, until in my late teens, terrified by her gray and puffy face, I brought her with me to the local YWCA where I swam for an hour several times a week. After I left for college, she continued to go to the pool with my father for a few more years, until he, in his midfifties, launched a start-up from a colleague's basement and began working late every night. She did love to garden and, in the warm months, spent hours outside weeding, pruning, and deadheading. But while this kept her flexible and surely relaxed her, her heart rate didn't budge. Her metabolism, only challenged by the occasional large meal, chugged along, constantly buffeted by the rich soup of free fatty acids endemic to a 5'4" woman carrying 220 pounds.

Her doctors monitored her carefully, but eventually she began to experience signs that her heart was failing. The mitochondria of her cardiac muscle cells had become less efficient at oxidizing fatty acids, their preferred fuel, despite the overabundance of them supplied by her ample adipose tissue. So they had shifted to rely more on glucose. This change, because it supplies less energy per reaction, overburdened her heart even more. The whole organ became enlarged, the pumping mechanism incompetent, and the passageways less elastic, pocked with scars and calcium deposits. She would halt, suddenly dizzy. "I need to sit down." She became breathless during the arduous trek from her first-floor bedroom to the dining room. And she was increasingly tired, dozing in her armchair or lying down suddenly—on four stacked pillows—for a midafternoon nap. Her cardiologist sent her to a cardiothoracic surgeon, who described her options: allow her weakened heart to peter out, probably within the next couple months, or have him replace her mitral valve. He seemed to take great glee in his description: She would be given general anesthesia, chilled down like a big fish on a block, and split open. They would attach her circulatory system to a heart-lung bypass machine, and he would go to work on the diseased organ, slicing out her valve and sewing in one from a pig.

The use of swine tissue in heart transplants began in the 1970s with the invention, by engineer Warren Hancock, of a flexible ring to which the valve could be sewn. Mechanical parts, while sturdy, require the patients to take anticlotting drugs for the rest of their lives, increasing their risk for bleeding events. Although a biologic device will wear out in fifteen years, it's usually preferred for older patients like my mother to avoid hemorrhages and strokes. Her apparatus, manufactured by Medtronic, was actually a byproduct of the pork raised for commercial consumption by companies such as Smithfield. After my mother came to from her eight-hour procedure, my brother, who'd flown to Boston from California, greeted her with a cheery "Hello, Miss Piggy!" For the next few years, we never lost the opportunity to make jokes about her porcine body part—besides her new nickname, we snorted and oinked at her, and gasped in shock at her cannibalism whenever bacon, ham, or other pork was served.

∞

I had contacted Michael Sturek, a professor of anatomy, cell biology, and physiology at the Indiana University School of Medicine, because I was investigating the health impact of the "chubby season," my name for the stretch that begins on Halloween and ends on our annual day of inertia, nursing hangovers, downing brews, and scarfing chips as we watch one of the venerable bowls—Fiesta, Rose, or Sugar. On average, the increase is just one pound, but one that sticks, contributing to long-term weight gain, and around five for those who are already overweight, according to multiple studies. Just how bad for us is this extended gluttony? How quickly does cardiovascular damage occur? Can it be reversed? And next year, what can we do to mitigate the impact of seasonal feasting? I'd read about a study Sturek had done that pretty much emulated the period of holiday blowouts, feeding sows a high-fat and high-calorie diet for nine weeks. The toll, even in this short period of overeating, was startling: the pigs not only got fat, they began to show symptoms of the metabolic syndrome, with worse cholesterol ratios, higher blood insulin levels, and thickening of the coronary arteries. But before you start declining party invitations, there was some encouraging news from another of Sturek's studies. In this one, done over twenty-four weeks, half the pigs were kept sedentary, while the other did daily workouts. While all the pigs gained weight, guess whose hearts, arteries, and circulatory systems looked healthy at the end of the study? Take-home: go ahead and eat the Snickers, pour the gravy, and pass the Christmas cookies, but don't take a break from physical activity and you can avoid negative health effects.

Sturek's interest in cardiovascular disease was deeply personal. Until he was two, his son Joshua, born in 1988, had been just like his older brother Jeffrey: same bottlebrush blonde hair, same impish grin, same indefatigable energy. Then Sturek and his wife began to notice odd little differences. Both boys ate ravenously, requesting second and third portions of their favorite food, Kraft macaroni and cheese, but while Jeff was stocky and well-muscled, Josh was stick thin and his ribs protruded. Both were even-tempered, but when Josh got tired, he had epic meltdowns that often ended in tears. And his breath was odd, with a fruity, even winy, scent to it.

In September 1991, shortly before his third birthday, the family's pediatrician gave the Stureks some bad news. Josh had type 1 diabetes. The toddler could go on to live a long and healthy life, she explained. But he would always need to eat carefully, get regular physical activity, monitor his blood-sugar levels, and inject insulin several times a day. Luckily, the Columbia, Missouri, couple was extraordinarily well prepared to take on management of a child's serious illness. Sturek had no squeamishness about medical procedures—he'd gotten a BA and MS in exercise physiology, before going on to earn a doctorate in pharmacology, and was then a researcher at the Dalton Cardiovascular Research Center at the University of Missouri. (When I ask him why the change from physical activity to pharmacology, he explains, "Exercise is actually a kind of drug because it acts on some of the molecular pathways and so forth that drugs do.") His wife, a certified public accountant, was a whiz at keeping records. But for Sturek, the diagnosis became a professional quest. Could he use his training to help his son? "It turns out that diabetes is a major risk factor for cardiovascular disease. So I started channeling more of our efforts into how diabetes causes such terrible heart disease."

The first task was to find a suitable research subject. The nonobese diabetic (NOD) mouse and the Bio-Breeding (BB) rat, both discovered in 1974, are the standard laboratory animals for diabetes research, but Sturek harbored concerns about experiments on rodents. "They are just very different from humans." Echoing Laurie Goodyear, he talks about how a mouse heart rate is five hundred beats per minute—and that doesn't change, even if you put it on a treadmill. For Sturek's projects, although they are more expensive and require more involved care, he decided to use our mammalian doppelgänger, the pig. "They're lazy, like a lot of human beings," Sturek says. "They like to just lie around." They are about our size, which means their organs are similar. Cardiologists viewing a video of a live heart angiogram can't tell them apart. "Half of them all guess pig, and half of them will guess human. It's that close," Sturek says. Pigs' resting heart rate, like ours, is about seventy-two beats per minute and increases with strenuous exertion. The similarities multiply when it comes to nutrition. Pigs and humans are two of the most flexible omnivores on earth, able to snarf up almost anything—and thrive. So it makes sense that our gastrointestinal systems—esophagi, stomachs, small intestines, and colons—are parallel. We also share many enzymes for the metabolism of nutrients, vitamins, and minerals, and even have very similar lipid ratios. "There is nearly complete agreement between humans and pigs in their dietary requirements," according to the 2000 book *Swine Nutrition*. But with all these likenesses, when it comes to being subjects for metabolic disease research, there's a catch. Unlike people, monkeys, rodents, and even cats, pigs don't naturally develop diabetes.

(Some scientists attribute this to the fact that pigs were domesticated as food stores for humans, so they evolved to flourish when being fattened.)

Sturek's first pig experiments were done in Yucatan Miniature Swine, a slender, gray breed known to be extremely docile, in which he'd induced diabetes by injecting them with alloxan, a drug that permanently inactivates the insulin-producing beta cells in the pancreas. The original Yucatan herd was brought to Colorado State University in 1960 with funding from the Kroc Foundation, a philanthropy begun by McDonald's founder Raymond Kroc, to support research on diabetes, from which he suffered and his daughter had died; arthritis; and multiple sclerosis. (Since then, purebred descendants of the charcoal-colored porkers have been acquired and commercialized by laboratory animal breeding companies such as Sinclair Research and Charles River Laboratories.) But Sturek still fretted. Were there differences in natural versus induced diabetes that might affect the results? How could he truly investigate the danger of heart disease in a body like his son's? The answer appeared almost by happenstance. In early November 2001, Sturek stumbled on a cranky letter to the editor in that week's edition of *Science*. The author, a feral animal ecologist, blasted an effort to remove introduced species from the Galápagos for failing to use the opportunity to collect data on them to better "know thy enemy." As an example, he cited a unique breed of feral pigs, on which his lab had accumulated thirty years' worth of data, that could drink seawater, gained weight more quickly than any other terrestrial creature, and developed diabetes. Sturek was gobsmacked. "I thought, my goodness, that's exactly what we need," he says. Sturek immediately contacted the writer, I. Lehr Brisbin, from the Savannah River Ecology Laboratory in Aiken, South Carolina.

"He said, 'We've been spending thousands and thousands of dollars of the government's money to try and make pigs diabetic in the laboratory to study them, and you're telling me you have an island full of pigs that are diabetic naturally?'" Brisbin recalls of that first telephone conversation. "I said, 'Please come visit.' And that was the start of one of the most remarkable collaborations I've had in my scientific career." The news, however, was not all good. Brisbin also told Sturek that the Ossabaw hogs were rapidly disappearing, under siege from the Georgia Department of Natural Resources (GDNR), which had essentially called permanent open season on them: "They are considered by many ecologists as the most devastating and hated vector of environmental destruction." It would be a race against time to save them.

Brisbin's pigs had an ancient pedigree. "On his final voyage to the New World, Christopher Columbus sailed from Spain to the Canary Islands and filled his boats with pigs," he explains. Not quite. According to historical records, just eight, from a breed that share Phoenician ancestry with their cousins, the Black Iberian pigs. But that eight, once established in Cuba, became many more. "They deliberately released these pigs on the islands in the Southeast as a source of food for the Spanish missions." That included Ossabaw Island, one of the dense network of barrier islands that shelter the Carolinas and Georgia from the battering Atlantic Ocean. There, the pigs went forth and multiplied in relative isolation for centuries, roaming over forty square miles of salt water marsh and upland covered with palm stands and hardwood forests. In summer and fall, they gorged; in winter, they virtually fasted.

"The Ossabaw hogs are truly omnivorous, they eat anything, but their major staple is the acorn crop," says Sturek. "The acorns drop in the fall, and those pigs are there munching those things down, but then that crop becomes exhausted. And there's the scarcity of food in the spring. They really go through these feast and famine cycles. . . . We hypothesize that really furthered evolutionary pressures for pigs that could pack away fat the best. So they develop these thrifty genes. And that's a big thing." Big because the same evolutionary pressure gave rise to a thrifty gene in that other highly successful omnivore, *Homo sapiens*—the same gene some scientists implicate in the global obesity epidemic, and which is connected to developing prediabetes, also called the metabolic syndrome.

"The metabolic syndrome is a whole suite of things that confer an advantage on free-living wild animals like pigs, or, as it turns out, like humans, who periodically face hard times and starve," Brisbin says. Among these is the ability to store fat in tiny droplets close to skeletal muscle mitochondria—just as do Iberian hogs. "The biochemistry of the fat, blood and tissue of the Ossabaw pig is different from other pigs," Brisbin explains. "And that's why it gets so fat, and stores the fat in its muscle tissue, and metabolizes it differently. And that, interestingly enough, makes it delicious. Ossabaw pigs win taste contests and food science studies." "The unique lipid-handling enzyme and hormone systems . . . allow them to rapidly and efficiently mobilize body fat reserves. . . . [But when] allowed high levels of caloric intake in captivity, obesity, insulin resistance, glucose intolerance, dyslipidemia, and hypertension develop. Ossabaw swine are the only miniature pigs to develop type 2 diabetes."[23]

In the wild, of course, the hogs don't get an opportunity to get life-style diseases: they're too active. To get an understanding of their movement patterns, I spoke to Kara Day, a biologist at the GDNR Wildlife Resources Division and game manager for the island. "They don't have a constant food source. And not only that, they don't have it all piled into a food pan where they can just waddle up and eat. They find an acorn here. They find a snail there. They find a snake over there. They've got to walk all over, be vigilant and ready to outrun a predator. So they're fast, and they're in shape. They wouldn't survive long if they weren't." But these are the good times. Day also describes the lean ones, and, despite her

23 I. Lehr Brisbin Jr. and Michael S. Sturek, "The Pigs of Ossabaw Island: A Case Study of the Application of Long-term Data in Management Plan Development," *In Wild Pigs: Biology, Damage, Control Techniques and Management*-SRNL-RP-2009-00869, ed. John Mayer and I. Lehr Brisbin Jr. (Aiken, SC: Savannah River National Laboratory, 2009), 367.

charge to eliminate them, admiration creeps into her voice. "Over the years, I've seen how hardy they are in their ability to survive such harsh environments. You see them with injuries that you can't believe they can sustain . . . missing a leg—their only native predator on the island is an alligator. . . . And sometimes they get snatched, or they'll get bitten, or they'll lose a leg, and you'll see them, they'll just bounce right back from that. It's amazing, really, that they can survive something like that and keep on keepin' on. You know, it's interesting to me that you see those hogs, once they're in captivity, they just look morbidly obese. But on the island, you rarely see any of that. And many times, what we see here is they look like they're just struggling, like they're skin and bones. They just look rough."

But the note of respect disappears when I ask Day to explain Georgia's policy on Ossabaw hogs. "There's a list of thirteen species in Georgia that are not protected by any game laws, or any kind of laws whatsoever, and the hog falls under that," she says. The wild pigs' voracity is their own worst enemy. In the late 1980s, the department had begun a campaign to control their numbers, removing over a thousand every year, but despite this, "discernible damage to other island resources continued to occur in the form of depredation of sea turtle nests and the rooting of oak hammock and salt marsh vegetation," Brisbin paraphrases a 1992 GDNR report in a paper. "During hunting season, when we have, say, our five deer hunts, we allow hunters to take as many hogs as they'd like while they're out there," continues Day. "If they want to shoot them all, go ahead, as many as you like. And then we also have hog-only hunts, so when hunters get selected for those hunts, and come out to the island, they can kill as many hogs as they want." In addition, the department pays a hog-control technician to live on the island. His only job is to reduce the colony.

Brisbin, with his new accomplice Sturek, concocted a swashbuckling plan to save the pigs, one that was pretty out of character for a couple of professors with two doctorates, hundreds of scientific articles, and several books between them. They would secretly breed an Ossabaw piglet colony in the bathtub of an old mansion on the island and rustle it to the mainland in the dead of night. "The state of Georgia said, we're going to exterminate the pig from Ossabaw Island because it didn't belong there," explains Brisbin. "And that infuriated us. We have no problems understanding that the pig roots up sea turtle nests—you have one unique and endangered form of animal eating another. And, you know, I can understand wanting to manage the pigs. But you don't have to exterminate them. So Sturek and I put this scheme together." There was also something more visceral behind Brisbin's defiance: revenge. He believed the state had double-crossed Eleanor "Sandy" Torrey West, a descendant of a wealthy Pennsylvania family that had bought the island in the 1920s, and, in the process, made a fool of him. West, with her second husband, Clifford Batement West, an artist, had enjoyed a bohemian lifestyle and, starting in the 1960s and continuing for decades, she regularly invited creative guests to the island during winter to paint, write, or compose music. Later, she founded the Genesis Project "to give young graduate students in biology and other fields a chance to live in the wild and study a unique ecosystem," says a 2016 article in *Gear Patrol*. Brisbin was the very first member. But as the land became more valuable and West's funds dwindled, she was strapped to pay the property taxes. She also wanted to ensure that the wilderness she loved continued intact into perpetuity. West arranged with the state of Georgia to purchase the entire island for half market value as a heritage preserve with a life tenancy. Before the deal was finalized in 1978, West asked Brisbin to review the sale documents. "And I looked over the contract. My [department head and another frequent visitor to the island] Gene Odom[24] looked over the contract. Everybody said, 'It's a good deal. It's just what you want.'

24 Eugene Odom (1913–2002), a University of Georgia faculty member, is considered to be the father of modern ecology, with the publication of his 1953 book, *Fundamentals of Ecology*.

And we were wrong. We got snookered by the state. . . . Because the state said, 'Okay, now we own the island. Hunt the pigs and the donkeys, and the cows gotta go.'"

To carry out the first part of their pig-saving plot, Brisbin enlisted Sandy West's help—not difficult, given that she was still smarting from the way the preservation deal had gone down and had even adopted a housetrained piglet injured by a hawk, who became her beloved pet Lucky. "'They used to go on walks around the island,' her grandson told the *New York Times* for her obituary, 'and then he would lie down on a riverbank, and she'd lean her head on his belly and read a book.'" Brisbin and his students did some hunting of their own—with tranquilizer guns and for pregnant sows. Once they had them, they moved them to an outdoor holding pen and waited for them to give birth. "[Piglets] are simply easier to move in large numbers than big pigs, and big pigs are nasty and want to bite you and knock you over." After each litter was born, they screened them for diseases—brucellosis, pseudorabies, and vesicular stomatitis, endemic to feral hogs throughout the United States. Some were born infected, but others were not, and so the scientist, his then-ninety-eight-year-old host, and team quarantined them in one of the bathtubs in West's twenty thousand square foot, pink stucco mansion.[25] Eventually, the piggy brood grew to ninety-seven squealing,

---

25 Ossabaw Island's current incarnation, a gracious mansion in a wilderness preserve, cloaks an ugly past. The Indigenous Gaules were burned out of their village by the Spanish in 1579. After a period of relative quiet as a hunting and fishing preserve for English settlers, in 1763, John Morel, a colonist, brought thirty slaves there to farm and timber. Later, indigo and then cotton plantations were established; during the 1800s, these were owned by four families and worked by at least 160 slaves who lived in cabins made of "tabby," a concrete made from crushed oyster shells and lime, three examples of which remain. After the Civil War, the island had a freedmen's settlement that established the Hinder Me Not African Baptist church. Many moved to the mainland community of Pinpoint after several devastating hurricanes in the late nineteenth century. The island was then purchased by the Torrey family, of which Eleanor West was a member, for $150,000. By the 1970s, the last remaining Black Ossabawans had abandoned the island.

straight-tailed, perky-eared, black youngsters, but until their blood had been tested and retested after a month and been proven to be absolutely clear of the three highly contagious diseases, they would have to stay put. "These were the standard regulations that farmers supposedly would have to adhere to if they were going to take their pigs across the state line to another state and establish breeding herds," explains Brisbin. "So it was nothing unusual, except that it's kind of silly in that every one of these diseases is rampant on the mainland anyway. So saying the Ossabaw pigs can't leave the island because they have these diseases—I mean, the mainland is full of them!"

Just twenty-six piglets eventually cleared the health hurdle. "We submitted all of their blood samples through our veterinarian from the University of Missouri to the state of Georgia laboratory testing and got these certificates saying that all the pigs were free of any infection," Brisbin says. Nonetheless, Georgia denied them permission to enter the mainland. Desperate, Brisbin applied to dock in nearby South Carolina, but this request was also refused. So he came up with a gutsy move that would get him labeled, he laughs, "a scoundrel, a troublemaker, and [author of] one of the most notorious kidnappings in Georgia wildlife history." In the very early morning on a spring day in 2002, Brisbin and his band of researchers and graduate students evacuated their charges on the *Eleanor*, West's barge, and drifted it the twenty minutes to the island's dock across the sound. "And they walked out of the barge onto an elevated chute, or a gang plank with fencing on the side, and marched right into an eighteen-wheeler tractor trailer. And their little feet never touched the soil of the state of Georgia." The truck traveled eleven hours to the University of Missouri, where they became the founders of Sturek's miracle pig colony.

"Once we got them back to the University of Missouri, they were in quarantine for about 180 days or so," says Sturek. "So it was a long road to really verify that we could keep these pigs on the mainland and so forth.

But the very interesting thing there is that we're the first team in about twenty years that took animals off that island." When Sturek was offered a position as a professor—eventually becoming department chair—at the Indiana School of Medicine Department of Cellular and Integrative Physiology, the pigs went with him. Sturek dedicated the next decade to establishing a breeding colony, demonstrating the Ossabaw's bona fides through dozens of proof-of-concept studies and encouraging their use by 140 different institutions, from the Mayo Clinic to Texas A&M University and Brown University. "[Initially,] we were a bit worried what would happen, because we spent a lot of money on this expedition and getting the pigs off the island. But when we did the studies—wow, it was amazing. And the fantastic thing is it, we've now published over one-hundred scientific articles on these pigs. And the [other institutions] can also document the prediabetes and insulin resistance, so it's really been confirmed very nicely. So hallelujah!" During this period, Sturek was supremely confident, crowing in a 2005 article in *Fortune*, "If you want me to blue-sky, five years from now our comparative medicine department will be studying a pig a day, and we'll be able to determine, say, which type of new stent helps prevent certain diseases in coronary arteries. Ten years from now we'll have lots of clues that will lead us toward preventing the majority of cardiovascular diseases." Among other endeavors, Sturek conducted what he calls "the coach potato project," in which they fattened up Ossabaws and then had them run on a treadmill. "If they're obese, and they start to exercise, it actually decreased their subsequent death from coronary artery disease, heart disease." By the end of the 2000s, it looked like the animal's potential contribution to diabetes and heart disease translational medicine was finally being recognized. In 2015 the National Institutes of Health allocated funding to the Swine Core to help Sturek further the use of the Ossabaw.

Instead, that year, the project stalled out and entered a tailspin. After approving a $308,148 annual budget for the enterprise, a joint

endeavor of Indiana University and Purdue University, which owns the
gene and which would breed and do research exclusively on Ossabaws,
the National Institutes of Health slashed the amount to $85,000
because of budget cuts, sequestration, and rising prices. At the same
time, Indiana University began to balk at the costs of caring for the
herd. "It put our unique animal resource in a financial death spiral,"
Sturek says. Meanwhile, the GNDR had finally succeeded in diminishing the island's herd which, according to Brisbin, had already been
tainted through crossbreeding. "Illegal hunters carrying pigs at night
in quiet boats [go] up into the salt marsh and release pregnant females
and others on it," Brisbin says. "So the original Ossabaw pig is now
mixed up with Eurasian wild boar hybrids. We don't even need DNA
[testing to know that], because the wild boar has striped piglets." Sturek's sixty pureblooded pigs were now probably the last ones on earth.

So Sturek engineered a second rescue, one that relied on the profit
motive rather than the budgetary whims of parsimonious universities
and unpredictable government funding. Together with two partners,
Mouhamad Alloosh, associate researcher professor, and James Byrd,
research technician, both also at the Indiana University School of
Medicine's Department of Cellular and Integrative Physiology, Sturek
chipped in about $130,000 in personal funds, sought an $800,000 bank
loan, and launched a start-up. The men struck a deal with Purdue University's Office of Technology Commercialization for the right to breed
and distribute the animals Sturek had discovered fifteen years earlier.
In 2018 Corvus BioMedical, LLC, opened the doors to a new, twelve-
acre facility in rural Montgomery County in west central Indiana with
dozens of pens, 140 hogs, and a tiny staff. Although they only made
$269,000 their first year, the founders are dreaming big again. Sturek,
Alloosh, and Byrd want to ratchet up production to one thousand pigs a
year and become a contract research organization "where we can conduct
a wide variety of medical research on these animals," Byrd explains in

a promotional video for the company. If everything goes according to plan, Sturek and his team hope to be the world's only source for purebred Ossabaw miniature hogs. And if things don't? Another tiny piece of the world's biological patrimony will quietly wink out.

∾

In the late 2000s, I made a radical career move: I shuttered our thriving public health agency to pursue fame and fortune as a writer. My first book was supposed to be a memoir of middle-aged awakening to my own self-centeredness set against the backdrop of a four-hundred-year-old Ecuadorian hacienda. The premise was I would learn to cook from the best home cook I knew, Carmen Quinaloa, an Indigenous woman who'd been employed there for almost twenty years. I sold the idea to an agent and then dragged my entire family for a month's stay in the Imbabura Province, close to the Colombian border. I spent my mornings in the kitchen with Carmen, then hiked the ancient Incan trails that riddled the area for an hour before lunch. In the afternoon, I had childcare duty, while Rafi roamed snapping photos. After we returned to the United States—with one case of salmonella (Rafi) and two of campylobacter (Gabi and Mariela), I wrote the first third of the book. I sent it nervously off to the agent. The story had changed a bit, because, well, when you spend so much time with people, reality. In particular, there was an episode involving Juancho, the hacienda's owner, and how he'd looked the other way about a fifteen-year-old girl's rape. My agent did not respond as quickly as I thought she would. Then came the email: the tone was very dark. She did not think the female readers seeking uplifting stories along the lines of *Eat, Pray, Love* would be pleased. Would I like to pitch her on another idea? Eventually I did, relegating Carmen's Kitchen to my virtual drawer of unfinished and rejected work.

But now, I keep thinking about a chapter draft—the one about Carmen's multiple moneymaking schemes to provide for her daughter, Isabela, and to even save for a rainy day. Of course, being from a small village high in the mountains, where people tend to be laconic, she didn't tell me any of this outright. The first clue was the chickens that swarmed the grand entrance to the hacienda. They were everywhere: weaving in and out of the whitewashed balustrades overhung with bougainvilleas that separated the drive from the wild area beyond; pecking their way around the empty, blue-tiled swimming pool; and, occasionally, disappearing inside the open front door of the little house set into the hill that rose to the east where Carmen lived with Isabela. Every day, she disappeared inside and came out with handfuls of corn kernels, which she scattered for the flock. "Why do you keep the chicken feed in your house?" I asked.

"Because it's mine. I bought it with *my* own money to feed *my* chickens." So this wasn't one of her tasks as cook, and since Rafi's aunt Micaela had died, the ostensible mistress of the household. Now I understood why her voice had glowed with pride when she pointed out the thickness of the shell and the orange tint of the yolk when she went out in the yard and returned with eggs to fry. The second clue was her cow. Several times a day, she headed off down the gnarled, cypress allée, telling me she had to tend to her *vaca*. I was slightly perplexed—why, on a dairy farm with hundreds of cows, who rotated pastures and amiably meandered to the barn at 4:30 A.M. and 4:30 P.M. to be milked, was there a need to tend a single herd member? One day, when we had gone to pick blackberries from the enormous bushes that edged the peach orchard, she detoured into the trunks and almond-shaped leaves and came back with a Guernsey on a lead. Carmen tied her to a tree and placed a plastic pail under her udder. Squirt, squirt, squirt. After hiding our pail of berries in the underbrush, we walked to the tiny town under the shadeless Andean sun. Carmen led me to a falling-down adobe building on the outermost street. She knocked on a peeling green door. "¿Señora?

¿Señora? Aquí estoy con la leche." The door creaked open. Inside was a very humble *viveres* (corner store). The owner took the pail into the back, returning with a clean one. She counted a couple of use-softened dollars into Carmen's palm. After we left, Carmen, who had first met me as the owner of a newspaper and knew that I owned a company in the States, commented, "A woman needs her own business so she can always take care of her children, no matter what happens. Am I right, Anastacia?"

But the crown jewel in her operation was the pig. After every meal, Carmen would fill a pail with slop from half-eaten plates, leftovers that had overstayed their welcome, and the remnants of the pots on the eight-burner stove. This tended toward carbohydrates—rice; *mote*, the Ecuadorian term for "hominy"; and potatoes, enlivened by a meat scrap, including, from time to time, a mouthful of a brother. There was no special chow and no concern about providing a balance of nutrients. We walked together to the mango grove, where, rooting under a tree heavy with fruit, was a large pig. It trotted over to greet us. "¿Y como le va al chanchito?" she said fondly, scratching behind its ears with a stick. Very well, obviously. Carmen's pig looked exceptionally healthy, with an alert face; a glowing, mottled black hide; and strong fore and hind legs. She poured the slop into a trough and the pig dug in. "Look how big he is already," she enthused. "When he's full-grown, I'll sell him at the market and finish paying off Isabela's computer."

Later during the visit, Carmen showed me how to prepare an Ecuadorian-style *pernil*, roasted pork haunch, a classic Latin American party dish. As do all good recipes, ours started with the search for the perfect ingredients. In this case, it meant a trip to Ibarra, the provincial seat, where there was a large municipal market, on the bus. The market took up several city blocks, and, like open-air markets everywhere—even when contained in concrete government buildings, it pulsed with people, goods, desire, and despair, all blanketed by the smells of frying street food, the slight rot of freshly butchered meat, acrid fish, heady flowers, honeyed fruit, and astringent vegetables. First, Carmen and I shopped for spices from a tapestry of red and gold tucked into a corner. After sliding the packets into her oilcloth market bag, we headed to *la señora de las carnes*, the one Carmen believed to have the best meat—from a pig raised as Carmen's was, outdoors and allowed to roam. Carmen whispered something to her, and she brought out a leg from the back, laying it gently across her forearms like a baby. Carmen pinched it and poked it, examining the white layer of fat and bulging blue-hued muscle under the thick skin. She nodded and peeled off a roll of bills. The woman wrapped the *pernil* in butcher paper, and we grabbed a taxi for the return trip, emitting contrails of dust along the town's dusty roads once we turned off the highway.

Although it was Thursday and the party was on Saturday, our preparations began that very day. Carmen washed and dried the pork and laid it in a shallow, rectangular pan. She handed me a fork. "Stab it all over. Make sure there's a good, deep hole every few centimeters." Meanwhile, she had collected a pile of *tomate de arbol*, a mild fruit that resembles an orange persimmon; red and white onions; garlic; sweet, red pepper; slender hot, red *ajíes*; sour oranges, lemons, and limes; olive oil infused with *achiote*; oregano; and cumin. She whirred up several blenderfuls, then poured it over the gravely wounded haunch, covered it in plastic wrap, and put it inside one of the three industrial-size refrigerators that lined the wall of the large kitchen. Our only task for the next day and a half was to flip it every four hours.

On Saturday, Juancho's five children, their partners, and assorted progeny began pouring in from Quito. They parked their cars—Jeeps and Mercedes—in the entrance and advanced, laughing and exclaiming, to the house. From the kitchen, where I was helping Carmen, I heard Juancho, standing at the door surrounded by his dogs, greet them, "Bienvenidos, hijos." The kitchen was awhirl with activity. Outside the door, Carmen had built a fire in the grill, where she was boiling *mote* and small potatoes. Inside, the pernil was slow-cooking in a 200 degree Fahrenheit oven. On the counter sat a large glass bowl of *cebolla curtida*, red pickled onion; pitchers of homemade juice; and Carmen's fiery *ají*, hot sauce. The two maids had been enlisted to set the tables and fetch drinks. When it was ready, the *hornado*, roasted pork, was so succulent it fell off the bone. Mixed with the mote and drizzled with the cooking juices, which Carmen had put into gravy bowls, it was irresistible.

The meal took place in both dining rooms—the children and teens seated at the intricately carved wooden table where we usually had our meals and the adults at a long marble one surrounded by upholstered chairs. I could hear shouts and laughter from the other room; my three girls had quickly been adopted by Isabela and the gang of cousins. Johnny Walker Black over ice clinked in the men's hands. The women giggled about a story told by one of Juancho's daughters-in-law. Outside, the sun sank behind the towering Andes, suddenly blanketing in shadow the main house, Moorish courtyard shaded by tall palms, and fifteenth-century monastery. I served myself another *poquito* of *pernil* and *mote*, spooned the cooking juices over it, and put a morsel in my mouth. I didn't chew, just let it fall apart on my tongue—the piquant sauce, the melting fat, and meat that tasted of sun, grass, and mountain arroyos. Perhaps by just holding it there I could stop time.

7

Backstroke-Swimming Roundworms

I looked everywhere, but couldn't find it. By process of elimination—personal care, no; vitamins, no; home health care, I don't think so; baby and child, maybe—it had to be here in first aid. I scoured the shelves. Nothing. It was 11:00 P.M., I was in dirty sweats, the first thing that had come to hand. Crap, crap, crap. I was going to have to ask. Slouching, I made my way to the disapproving woman with a bindi stocking shelves.

"Excuse me. Um. Could you tell me where the pinworm medicine is?" I felt her mentally jump back a yard.

"First aid, bottom shelf. Next to the lice treatment," she said coldly. I flinched. Unfortunately, I was intimately familiar with that, too. I returned, squatted, and peered into the bottom shelf. There, pushed out of view, were a couple green-and-white boxes of Reese's pinworm medicine with FOR THE ENTIRE FAMILY emblazoned across a pop-out yellow stripe. I cleaned out their entire stock of three, paid without meeting the cashier's eyes, and sped home. Less than an hour had passed since, after showering and putting on her pajamas, Mariela had said to me, "Mama, my butt is itchy." But I knew, even without the recommended home evaluation, which calls for getting up in the dead of night, shining a flashlight on your child's anus, and looking for tiny lady worms releasing clouds of microscopic eggs—exactly what was wrong—and what to do about it.

"Everyone line up! Deworming time!"

"Why do I have to take it if Mariela's the one who has them?" Gabriela grumbled.

"Because they are highly contagious. You don't want pinworms, do you?" We all slugged down our carefully measured dosages of the chalky, yellowish liquid, even my mother. I hoped it wouldn't interfere with any of her dozens of medications and supplements. Then it was time for deep cleaning. All of Mariela's bedding, clothes, and stuffed animals. All the towels, mats, and washcloths in the bathrooms. I bleached the toilets, sinks, bathtub, and shower stall. I scoured surfaces, doorknobs, and light switches all around the house. Tomorrow I would do the same. (Sometimes I think these childhood plagues are just invented to smack some housewifery into those of us who shirk it.) But that was just the cleanup of the material world. Now came the hard part: telling anyone with whom she'd had close contact that she had worms. Which in Mariela's case was her entire gymnastics club, with which she practiced for four or five hours four days a week. (Is there a better recipe for a pinworm infestation than a group of school-age girls taking turns running their hands over a variety of equipment, adjusting their wedgie-prone leotards—per regulations, no undies—and then happily munching their bags of Goldfish and apple slices at snack time?) What should I do? Send out a group email?

Mariela would feel like a pariah. It was bad enough that we sometimes struggled to pay the monthly bill, uniforms, and meet fees, and on several occasions, had kept her home while the rest of the team flew to Florida or the Bahamas. Getting her into the sport had originally been Rafi's idea, who'd been a gymnast in Cuba, where clubs are state-sponsored. "Gymnastics?" I'd asked foolishly. "Isn't that expensive?" But now she'd been part of the club for several years and, since we homeschooled, it was an important source of social interactions for her. Telling the other families that our daughter, with her Target shoes and sisters' hand-me-downs, had a roiling parasite infection and most probably had given it to their daughters made me feel defeated, gross, and embarrassed. Her too, I gathered, when I informed her it was our responsibility to share the information with the club. "Nooo!"

∽

I was one of those kids who read everything, even the back of the tooth-paste tube. If it had words on it, I needed to know what they said. If there were pages, I was compelled to flip through them. Which is why, at the age of six, I was well-acquainted with the contents of *Better Homes & Gardens*, *Women's Day*, and *Family Circle*, the 1970s women's magazines my mother subscribed to. While I religiously worked my way through the articles, mostly peppy how-tos on everything from decorating and cooking to fashion, what I really pored over were the ads. These mostly fell into two categories, cleaning and beauty products, but there was one that, no matter how often I saw it, arrested me in horror. It was black and white and depicted a mass of writhing tiny, white worms. DOES YOUR CHILD HAVE PINWORMS? the headline demanded. The body copy explained how the tiny parasites were common, extremely contagious, and could be cured with the advertiser's medicine. In me, it triggered a weeks-long obsession with staring deeply into the toilet before flushing and trips to my parents' bedroom to request a maternal inspection. I never actually got them, but they occupied a top spot on my list of childhood terrors.

As far as human parasites go—and of about 370 total, 300 are worms—pinworms are as harmless as you get. They've been hitching a free ride with us for at least ten thousand years—their eggs were found in petrified person poop in Utah's Danger Cave (so-named because, in the 1940s, a boulder crashed down near the entrance while some arche-ologists were at work there), along with two other species, the tape and thorny-headed worms. Other analyses of ancient Indigenous excrement have upped the number of infecting species, and, fascinatingly, shown that hunter-gatherers were far less prone to the parasites than agriculturalists. (Which makes sense when you think about it. Those on the move traveled in small groups and did their business in a variety of locations. This would make it harder for parasites to enter a new host.) Pinworms are exquisitely well adapted to us, spending only a nominal time outside of our bodies in their life cycles, and—probably to maintain us in prime condition for feeding (they swallow miniscule quantities of epithelial cells and bacteria)—do not generally lacerate tissue, as do hookworms, tapeworms, and other roundworms. (Lest I've painted them as too innocuous, chimpanzees infected with human pinworms often die.) Inside us, they do the things that living things like to do, including worm sex, between a shrimpy male with a special vulva-opening prong called a spicule and a female, who is generally two to four times his size, although herself no longer than the smallest sewing pin, the lill, used by crafters for beads and sequins and by entomologists to display their insect collections. After copulation, he dies. She gestates, then, reminiscent of the majestic birthing exodus of Antarctic penguins, sets out, alone, full of her progeny, on a treacherous nighttime journey through the large intestine. (The slight drop in body temperature during sleep is her cue to embark.) Half crawling, half swimming—the complex postures she assumes are called eigenworms by mathematicians, the mother-to-be propels herself forward by thrashing back and forth as the passageway rhythmically squeezes and releases. If she is unlucky, she is momentarily caught in a violent storm—the two or three daily "mass action'" contractions, which load feces into the firing position. At the end of her arduous five-foot trek, she emerges at the anus to lay ten thousand tiny, itchy eggs. And then she dies, her evolutionary mandate to reproduce fulfilled.

When I ask Jessica Hartman, assistant professor of biochemistry at the Medical University of South Carolina (MUSC), how much exercise parasitic worms get inside their hosts, she is taken aback. "I thought you couldn't ask a new question when you said it was a crazy question. . . . But that was a new question." Can you speculate? I press. "I really have no idea," she says. But it makes perfect sense to me—Hartman, along with a few far-flung collaborators, including Ricardo Laranjeiro, a postdoctoral associate at the Rutgers School of Arts and Sciences, studies the impact of physical activity on *Caenorhabditis elegans*, a free-living roundworm. Just as she explains to me how her one-millimeter-long subjects move about in their preferred habitat, rotting vegetation and mucky soil, I figure she might know something about their extremely mobile, parasitic cousins. No such luck. Nor do online accounts of the creatures' natural history, although I am delighted to learn that, when they are seeking temporary hosts for dispersal, the larvae balance on their tails and do group waves, just like sports fans. Similar to laboratory mice and rats, *C. elegans* is a model species. Scientists have mapped out their entire genome—the very first multicellular creature to be so honored, as a matter of fact—and turn to them time and time again for experiments. They are the only animal with a complete "connectome," a diagram of its entire neurological system, making them ideal for research on diseases and conditions that affect the brain, aging, and cognitive function.

One of the places this is happening is at the Driscoll Lab at Rutgers, where a couple dozen scientists, technicians, and support staff carry out all sorts of healthspan studies. "*C. elegans* has a lot of advantages for genetic manipulation. They only live for two to three weeks. So you can follow the effects of exercise throughout the entire lifespan," Laranjeiro explains. "They are also transparent, which makes it very easy to image cells in vivo, including single neurons, which is pretty much impossible to do in mammals." But before he and his colleagues could see what kind of impact regular, intense movement had on *C. elegans* mitochondria, Laranjeiro would have to figure out how to get them to follow a fitness regimen. This was not an easy feat. In the lab, the animals spend their days lolling on delicious *E. coli*–coated agar held in six-centimeter-wide petri dishes. To get them off their duffs, Laranjeiro transferred them to a dish topped off with a watery solution. "They start to swim. And during the swimming, they move much faster than during the crawling. But we had to prove that they were actually exercising, so we had to show that they were consuming more energy during the swimming. . . . My first paper, the one in *BMC Biology* in 2017, was for just a single exercise session of a ninety-minute swim, to show that the reaction to that session is pretty similar to what happens in mammals. . . . We measured, for example, mitochondrial oxidation levels in the muscle. And then we also looked at glucose metabolism and fat metabolism. And we saw that the fat reserves in the muscle seem to be the main source of energy for that ninety-minute swim." (Previous experiments, which had left the critters to tread water indefinitely, had established that after an hour and half to two hours the worms become so tired they have to do a dead man's float every few minutes.)

From there, Laranjeiro at Rutgers and Hartman at MUSC both began to work out the ideal protocol to create fit worms without overtaxing them so they could research the impacts of longer-term physical activity. They came up with slightly different approaches, which Hartman teasingly chalks up to their respective reverence for the weekend. Laranjeiro's, which he calls the 3 + 3 + 2 + 2 protocol, had the animals doing laps for three ninety-minute sessions on days one and two of adulthood, then two sessions on days three and four. Handily, the protocol was done by Friday. Hartman, however, wanted to cover the worms' entire reproductive lives, so her regime was twice daily sessions for six days—obligating researchers to trudge into work on Saturdays. "My protocol ends up having twelve sessions over six days," Hartman says. "His protocol ends up having ten sessions over four days. So they're pretty comparable. . . . In general, he and I both observed really fascinating benefits from the exercise." For one, the nematodes were noticeably buff. "When you raise them in liquid, they are thinner and longer than their counterparts that live on the agar," Hartman says. "So it really changes their whole physiology to grow up that way. . . . And even early on, [Ricardo] and I both noticed that they just moved around a lot more than the control worms at the end of the exercise sessions. So these were just more active animals, which is so cool. It's such a simple, small organism, and it seems that they really do have these benefits."

I ask both scientists to describe the changes they saw. "The mito-chondria were just maintaining their networks much better," Hartman says. "These are very complex organelles, constantly changing their shape based on energetic needs. So they might become more fused to where you have like one big mitochondria, all connected together. Or they might fragment, and then you have a bunch of little mitochondria. And you can imagine there would be benefits to both. So if you need to get rid of some old dysfunctional pieces of mitochondria, you would want them to be in smaller pieces. And so in that case, breaking apart might be just a normal part of quality control. But other groups have shown that when mitochondria fuse, that they're more efficient at making energy. So fusion is generally thought of to be a good thing. . . . And they're in these beautiful lines, like you can see where the mitochondrial networks mirror the organization of the muscle fibers."

These changes were long-lasting and forestalled the deterioration associated with aging. "If you look at young animals, and in the muscle cells, the entire muscle cell is covered by a mitochondrial network," Laranjeiro says. "And then over time, the network starts breaking down, there's a lot of gaps, the mitochondria start to [become] round rather than being more filamentous. That's the normal progression of the aging phenotype. So what we saw was that the exercised worms maintained the mitochondrial network much better throughout their lives, [although it] eventually starts to decay. But it lasts for a long time." Hartman seconds that. "We saw that, in controls, as they aged, those mitochondria became more sparse. They were just fewer and more separated from one another. So they were fragmented. . . . If you look at older animals, it gets worse and worse. But then our exercised animals maintained those healthy, young-looking networks longer into life."

The organelles from fit worms were able to generate more energy than their unexercised counterparts. "We also look at the function of the mitochondria, not just how they look, but if they work better. For that, we use the oxygen consumption rate assays, where you can see if they are consuming oxygen and at what levels, and we saw that in the exercised worms, once again, the mitochondria are healthier. They can respond to different stressors and produce the oxygen consumption rates at a much healthier level," Laranjeiro says. Hartman explains, "In animals, the majority of oxygen that's consumed is going through the mitochondrial respiratory chain. So we can use this oxygen consumption to say something about mitochondrial function. And so we did a laborious experiment, where we looked under a microscope and looked for the fragmented phenotype we were seeing pop up in older animals. We picked only those animals with fragmented mitochondria. And [compared them to] animals that had more networked, fused mitochondria. And we saw a big difference in how much oxygen consumption there was. So we were able to say that, indeed, when we see this fused mitochondria in a beautiful network, they are also functioning at a higher level as well." Physical activity increased the worms' mitochondrial "spare capacity," the difference between its ability to create energy at the basal, or resting, rate, and its maximal respiration rate, and, at least in muscle cells, reduced the number of reactive oxygen species, the molecules that cause inflammation.

But that's not all. In-shape worms are not only better able to deal with internal toxins—inflammation and abnormal accumulations of protein, such as you might see in Alzheimer's, they are also better able to deal with external ones. The scientists' experiment examined whether the cells of exercised worms are more resistant to arsenic and rotenone, a pesticide. "The most exciting moment, I think, during the beginning of that project was when I had worms that had exercised for the six days. And then at the end of that twelve-session protocol, I put them in different doses of arsenic. Arsenic is still a really common drinking water contaminant in many places, including the US, but it's much worse in other places globally. And what I found was, I waited twenty-four hours with them in the arsenic, and then I looked at the plates, and all of the control worms were dead. I mean, you know, they couldn't survive it. But my exercised animals were swimming happily. Wow." Hartman believes their findings are a start to answering such questions as whether running in urban areas, which is known to increase your exposure to air pollution since you regularly spend time outside breathing heavily, may not necessarily be as toxic as for sedentary people. "If you're an exercise-conditioned person, are you going to respond differently?"

The pair's *C. elegans* have even had their fifteen minutes of fame. In December 2018 Laranjeiro sent thousands of tiny cosmonauts tucked into small sacks holding a liquid culture laced with freeze-dried *E. coli* rations to the International Space Station. Because he and his colleagues didn't think they could presume on astronauts to monitor the nematodes' lap swimming, there was no exercise protocol, although some collaborators at Texas Tech University are working on some microfluidic devices for future missions. Instead, Laranjeiro looked at the impact of space travel on neurons. The results may give pause for anyone considering blasting off for an extended period of time. "In our lab, we have shown that the neurons can release some big vesicles that contain trash and mitochondria, which we think it's a way to get rid of some damaged mitochondria and some other damaged proteins. And those vesicles are released to the tissues outside the neuron. So in the worms that stayed on earth, those vesicles seem to be degraded, and there's no accumulation [of trash] in the surrounding tissues. But the ones that went to space, there was an accumulation of that fluorescent trash. It seemed like the neighboring tissues were not able to degrade those vesicles efficiently. So that's why we suggest that, especially for long-term spaceflight, that might create some functional problems in the neurons." Laranjeiro isn't drawing any definitive conclusions, but he definitely thinks the subject should be studied more.

∾

My choice of ballet schools didn't go over well with Rafi. First, there was the matter of the location: the third floor of a rundown brick building that housed a street-front shoe store with a bright red door above which an equally bright-red sign screamed THE CENTER FOR MARXIST EDUCATION. (The center was on the second floor to the right. To the left was a tailor whose mannequins and racks of handiwork lined the staircase like weary bystanders.) Then there was the fact that the class size was teeny—Esmerelda, her good friend, a pair of sisters, and a quiet boy named Luke—and that the padded latex floor seemed to be held together with duct tape. The school wasn't uptight about cleanliness. And as for dress—leotard and tights, fine! T-shirt and sweats, also fine! Glitter? Boas? Go for it! But Rafi's objections didn't stand a chance alongside the fact that the prices were incredibly reasonable, that it served the diverse neighborhood, and every student danced in at least one performance a year.

The studio occupied most of the third floor. At the far end, overlooking the busy street, was a changing area with cubbies. Coming up the steps, you emerged into a hall so narrow that the parents sitting in the line of plastic chairs against the stairwell bannister could practically touch the practice area doorway—blocked off with a heavy tan curtain—with their fingertips. Although we were asked not to, we often peeked through it, eager to see our offspring assume one of the five positions or struggle to obey the instructor, a former company dancer, as he barked "Plier! Glisser! Éntendre!" As we waited, we chatted, at first about our children, then about the details of our lives, and soon about more personal things. I'd taken a liking to Luke's mother, who had a calm, kind face and wore scarves made of hand-loomed textiles. Sometimes Luke's father, a stocky man with very thick glasses, would drop him off. On those days, Madeleine appeared, looking slightly harried, toward the end of class to bring him home. When I learned that this involved two bus rides and two subway trips and that they only lived a mile or so from us, I offered to give Luke a ride, which became our twice-weekly ritual. I didn't think too much about it. I often tried to step up with other friends who didn't have vehicles, either because they were environmentalists; ardent cyclists; couldn't afford repairs, insurance, and gas; or, as was most common, all three. But one day when Madeleine was on drop-off duty, I said something to the effect that I admired their commitment to living car-free. Madeleine smiled and told me it wasn't a matter of choice. Her partner was legally blind, and it was either use public transportation or be the only chauffeur in a busy family of five. "He had river blindness," she said. "Growing up in Louisiana. It was common there." I thought, but didn't say, how much I admired the effortlessness with which they navigated this permanent challenge.

You don't catch river blindness, as you might think, by immersing yourself in unclean waters. The name comes from the British Empire Society for the Blind which, in the 1950s, was trying to raise funds for the sub-Saharan victims of *kru kru* or *craw craw* and didn't think the African words would have much traction with the English public. It rebranded the disease, emphasizing its spread by the blackflies that breed in fast-moving rivers and streams. Onchocerciasis, its medical designation, begins in an infected human, under whose skin teem millions of worms, possibly up to 150 million for someone with a severe case, in the first of three larval stages. Along comes a lady fly with the arthropod equivalent of PMS: she needs a blood snack to lay her eggs, which she will do, on average, two to three times during her lifetime, according to entomologist Elmer W. Gray at the University of Georgia. She nips and sucks, in doing so vacuuming up an infusion of larvae. These spend a week maturing to second and then third stages inside her, at which point, during her next preovulatory prowl, they are transferred back to a human host, and the cycle begins again. Once deposited, the larvae create a fibrous nodule, visible under the skin and often in the torso or head, where they mature for six months to a year. The adult female is, frankly, a beast. Fourteen to twenty-four inches long, she spends most of her time coiled up in the nodule, while the much smaller males move hither and thither. (Her interest in them is minimal; their presence is not even required for reproduction.) The stately dame lives for ten to fifteen years—yes, you read that correctly—and lays 500–1,500 microscopic prelarvae daily. These tiny filaments are so small they pass through tissues and disperse throughout the body under the skin, where they cause itching so infernal it drives people to scar themselves. Similarly, worms can penetrate the eyes, where they can gravely irritate the cornea, causing vision loss. River blindness voyaged to the New World with the transatlantic slave trade, where it became endemic, especially in Central and South America. Although huge strides have been made in eliminating the disease—congratulations, Colombia, Ecuador, Mexico, and Guatemala—an estimated eighteen million people still carry the worms, almost all of them in Africa. Their lives, like that of my friend's family, may be irrevocably limited by disfigurement in a region where simple survival is already a struggle.

Pinworms and the invaders that cause river blindness are both members of a scarily populous branch of worms, the nematodes, or roundworms, which may have up to one million species and are no slouches when it comes to reproducing. Scientists estimate that there are fifty-seven billion nematodes for each one of us. (The other major branch is flatworms, to which belong tapeworms and flukes.) Roundworms are both free living, inhabiting practically all environments—fresh and salt water, ocean floors and mountaintops, where they dine on micro-organisms, debris, and other tinier worms—and parasitic, inhabiting and consuming from inside all types of plants and animals. Although the common pinworm does not carry disease or damage its host, this is not true of its fellow parasitic roundworms. The eggs or early stage larvae are often spread in soil and their development entails gruesome odysseys through the liver, heart, and lungs, where juvenile worms may be coughed up and swallowed or burrow their way back through the intestinal wall. Others, like the species that causes river blindness, are disseminated through a secondary host. In addition to biting insects, this includes snails, who pollute fresh water with larvae that then enter humans. Their impact is colossal. In 2020 the World Health Organization (WHO) estimated that 1.5 billion people, roughly a quarter of the world's population, have infections, primarily in sub-Saharan Africa, Asia, and the Americas.

Antonio Montresor, who runs the community intervention program of the WHO's Department of Control of Neglected Tropical Diseases, has immense respect for parasitic worms. "They are more intelligent animals than malaria. They don't want to kill the host because the host is where they get food, they get shelter, they get heating—everything. So, if they replicate—because every worm can produce thousands of worms—and if all these eggs hatch in the human body, they will kill the host. So they have to stay in the soil for a period to mature and then infect another person." Of course. I have been reading about roundworms and talking to helminth, parasitic worm, experts for a while, but no one has explained why their reproduction always involves at least one phase outside the human body. Until now. Wily critters! Of course, as Montresor points out, this extracorporeal phase makes for a lot of environmental dissemination and is a reason why children, who often play in the dirt, especially in warmer climates, make up more than half of all worm infections and are the ones who suffer the most harm. "This parasite, of course, competes for vitamins, for micronutrients, for everything. So, if [worms are combined with poor-quality food], "this can cause a significant nutritional impact." Montresor's program distributes biannual deworming medicine to teachers. This doesn't permanently eliminate the plague, but it does interrupt the worms' life cycle enough to keep the disease burden to a minimum, so that children's physical and cognitive growth isn't affected. Since 2008, when the WHO established its soil-transmitted helminth control program, the percentage of children treated in endemic areas has climbed from 10 to 60—more than 650 million children in 2019, enough of a success that they are now trying to expand to another vulnerable group, women of reproductive age. Younger women face an anemia and B-vitamin deficiency trifecta: persistent, low-level blood loss from parasitic infections; menstruation; and malnutrition. "There is no chance that this girl is in good health," Montresor says, and if she gets pregnant, "the child will be born malnourished. . . . But what I think is most interesting [about this situation] is the cost of the intervention. Because these drugs are quite old and extremely cheap. On the market, you can buy one tablet of albendazole for two cents. That means that for two dollars, we can treat one hundred children . . . And because we use existing infrastructure, twenty thousand teachers who distribute it for one hour every six months, this intervention is very near to zero cost."

I ask Montresor to describe exactly how people get infected. First, of course, some worms pierce the feet, hands, or other parts of the body. This is not, as I had imagined, through tiny cuts and cracks in the sole, which, in someone who regularly goes unshod, is thick and tough. "The eggs, they go on the grass leaf and when the child or the person passes, they basically drop down" on top of the foot, between the toes, where the skin is softest, Montresor explains.

"So a sandal or a flip-flop won't protect you?" I ask him.

"No," Montresor scoffs. Besides, he kindly points out, purchasing shoes for a family in low-income countries would not only present logistical difficulties, it would be orders of magnitude more expensive than the regular deworming. A whole other category of helminths kicks off their infestation by being swallowed, for which life in the Global South presents many opportunities. "If the child is working in the sand or on the floor, and the floor is contaminated, for example, or outside in a garden, then the eggs can stay on the fingernails. If you don't wash your hands before you eat, you can ingest the eggs." They can also persist in food itself, which is why tourists are advised to avoid salads. "So basically, when in tropical countries, it's better to eat vegetables that you can peel or you can cook." Not only can crops be contaminated by infected field workers, in some regions, fresh or inadequately processed human feces is used as fertilizer; for example, Montresor says, in Vietnam, China, and Cambodia. "Human feces should be at least composted for a period to [get rid of] the eggs—so basic sanitation and food habits are essential."

There is a breathtakingly easy solution to ending soil-transmitted helminth infections: the latrine. Yet even this piece of rudimentary infrastructure, critical to containing eggs and larva and preventing reinfection—is often beyond the reach of those who most need them. "Building latrines is quite expensive," Montresor says. "Normally, it is not something that should be done by the government, but should be done by the individuals. But if the individual has sufficient resources, first of all, they want to have shelter, and they want to have food. And then they want to have a mobile phone. And then, maybe, they will buy a motorbike and then, finally, a latrine." I'm puzzled. Why do latrines have to be individual decisions, if they are so crucial to public health? American cities eliminated many of these sorts of fecal-oral route diseases by engaging in large public work projects—first potable water, and then, quickly afterward, when usage soared, sewers. Today urbanites can install toilets for a few hundred dollars and about $250 a year for sewage thereafter. (Although the rural poor are still left shouldering the burden of their own septic systems—which can cost thousands to install and a couple hundred a year to maintain.) In fact, there is now a movement afoot to reinvent the toilet, spurred in part by a 2011 Bill & Melinda Gates Foundation grants program to create affordable, off-the-grid sanitation systems. One of these, Loowatt, now being piloted in Madagascar, South Africa, and the Philippines, has created home toilets under which waste is sealed in a polymer film after each use and stored in a barrel, the contents of which are regularly collected and turned into biofuel or fertilizer.

If you find yourself, as I did, wondering how it's possible you didn't know what a blight parasitic worms are for humanity, and most tragically, millions of children, it's not by accident. Soil-transmitted helminths make up the largest proportion of what are called neglected tropical diseases, an offshoot of the field of tropical medicine, one of the many altruistic-sounding props invented to maintain the British Empire. By the late eighteenth century, vexed from the loss of the American colonies, the British turned their attention east and south, using a combination of administrative control, military might, and economic clout to dominate India, a large swath of Africa, and most of Southeast Asia, as well as parts of Asia, the Caribbean, and South America, acquiring tens of millions of square miles of land and hundreds of millions of new subjects. This shifted the center of British territory to the equator where warm, humid climates predominate year-round, allowing soil and insect-borne diseases to flourish. (In case you feel you've dodged a bullet, cooler zones, where people tend to congregate indoors when the temperature drops, are perfectly suited for the exchange of viral upper respiratory infections, such as colds, influenza, and COVID-19.) Employees of the Colonial, Foreign, and India Offices; representatives of British trading companies; explorers; missionaries; settlers; and sometimes their families descended on all corners of the empire, falling prey to a host of new maladies.

"Tropical medicine goes back to the boots-on-the-ground colonial era, where you have European colonial powers, being physically present in colonized lands, and of course, encountering diseases that are new to them," says Arianne Shahvisi, a brilliant cross-disciplinary philosopher at the Brighton and Sussex Medical School in England. To give you an idea of her intellectual firepower, she studied natural sciences at Cambridge, then did two master's, one in astrophysics, the other in the philosophy of physics, then returned to Cambridge for a doctorate in philosophy, all the while tossing off extravagantly precise journal articles and evocative book reviews and personal essays for *Prospect*, *New Statesman*, and the *London Review of Books*. But, of course, over Zoom, she comes across as just plain nice. "It's very difficult to colonize a country if you're ill. And so tropical medicine came out of the need to keep colonizers healthy, . essentially. And also, I suppose, to keep colonized peoples healthy to some extent as well, if you were reliant upon them as a source of cheap or free labor." In fact, the specialty did not truly emerge until the end of the nineteenth century, when Patrick Manson, a Scottish doctor, founded the London School of Hygiene & Tropical Medicine with a donation from an Indian philanthropist. Manson had spent eighteen years in China and Formosa (present-day Taiwan), and had figured out the life cycle of the worm that causes elephantiasis, a grotesque swelling of the lower appendages. The first set of tropical diseases to be cracked were the ones that affected rich and poor indiscriminately—malaria, yellow fever, and the aforementioned elephantiasis, all dispensed by the impudent mosquito. But the ones that were linked to poor sanitation and "hygiene" (this term makes me cringe; it's hard to be hygienic if you've been forced off your native land by colonizers and are living in a shack) were mostly confined to Indigenous populations—and were largely ignored.

After triumphantly spearheading the reduction of malaria, tuberculosis, and, much later, HIV/AIDS, country-specific tropical disease research declined. "You no longer have that drive to keep colonizers healthy, because they're not there anymore, right?" Shahvisi says. "Colonialism is still a feature of the world in which we live, [but] in a very different way—very much at a distance. And so there's no longer really any motivation to be interested in diseases which prevail in particular regions or that affect particular people. . . . If you live far away, you don't need to worry about it. . . . The other important point to make here is, these are not puzzling diseases, they're not scientific mysteries. They're very controllable. They're very treatable. They're eradicable. The point is, we're not putting the resources into doing this. And yeah, I think it's because, as you say, they're at the bottom of the pile in terms of how much of a threat they actually pose to you, or me, or to other people living in world regions where there's money and power." In 1977 the American medical researcher Kenneth S. Warren assumed leadership of the Rockefeller Foundation's Medical Sciences Division and, for eight years, funded a network of research laboratories to study what he called the "great neglected diseases"—deliberately choosing the term *neglected* as a public relations shock technique, an effort that resulted in hundreds of specially trained scientists and published papers. After that, the United Nations took up the mantle. Although there are dozens of neglected tropical diseases, seventeen have been singled out as being especially devastating for the world's poorest inhabitants, who, as the WHO website notes, live "in remote, rural areas, urban slums, or conflict zones." About half—cysticercosis, guinea-worm disease, echinococcosis, foodborne trematode infections, lymphatic filariasis, river blindness, schistosomiasis bilharziasis, and soil-transmitted helminthiases—are caused by parasitic worms, spread through ingesting the eggs, walking barefoot where larvae are present, contact with water that has been poisoned by infected snails, or by the bite of a carrier insect.

Shahvisi argues that the term *neglected tropical diseases* is disingenuous, intended to further distance us from their victims and to erase the Global North's historic role in creating or perpetuating the conditions in which the diseases thrive. "If you look at a map of disease burden, you do see that it is concentrated on the continent of Africa, in sub-Saharan Africa, in particular. But that's got nothing to do with how hot it is, right? I mean, Australia is a very hot country, right? . . . And yet, of course, its contribution to global disease burden is very small, because it has a good-functioning health system. And it's health systems that correlate with high disease burden, not something to do with temperature. There is this sense that we have of the Global South as a place of sickness, as a place of diseases, a place of disorder, and inefficiency. And people being unable to do things right. . . . And it really is harder for somebody to get the health care that they need. But there are reasons for that. There's a whole history, and that history just kind of gets snipped out." Instead of *neglected tropical diseases*, Shahvisi advocates the forthright phrase *diseases of poverty*.

The course for the fourteenth summer Olympics marathon, on September 10, 1960, wound through the streets of Rome, passing sites such as Piazza di Campidoglio, the Caracalla Baths, and the Appian Way, like a whirlwind tour of the city's ancient architecture. After an early evening start to avoid the heat of the day, a scrum of almost seventy runners finished in the dark under the Arch of Constantine, where, for the first time in Olympic history, two Black African runners had taken the lead. In the final five hundred yards, one pulled ahead: a bone-thin, last-minute entrant from Ethiopia, twenty-eight-year-old Abebe Bikili. He had set a new world record and had done so barefoot—because Adidas, the supplier, had run out of his size. Today, many races have a small contingent of no-footwear athletes, or those wearing shoes with little sole or separate compartments for each toe, inspired by the 2009 bestseller *Born to Run* by Christopher McDougall or an influential 2010 study of foot-strike patterns by evolutionary biologist Daniel Lieberman. But our glorification of barefoot running divorces it from its original context, which is destitution. Many of the runners who brought it to world attention—Bikili, and later Zola Budd and Legla Laroupe—were from small African villages. Their families likely could not afford to build latrines, purify drinking water, or purchase shoes. Bikili, who grew up in a tiny highland village, Jato, fifty miles from Ethiopia's capital, Addis Ababa, spent his childhood herding goats and stopped going to school at the age of twelve. For fun, he played *genna*, an ancient game performed with root balls and eucalyptus sticks— a friendly town match has become part of the Ethiopian Christmas tradition. The playing field can be as large as the area between rival villages. This naturally required a lot of shoeless running in wide-open spaces. Exhilarating! But also a public health hazard. Children who play barefoot are exposed to the larva of large roundworms, hookworms, and whipworms, all of which enter through the skin. Highland Ethiopians have an infection rate of about 20 percent, according to a 2013 study. It is profoundly disrespectful of the desolation these parasites cause to not consider this widespread human reality in our Global North debates on how not wearing shoes affects jogging injuries. Especially when it can be mitigated by medication that, per child, costs pennies.

∽

The human body does not take invasions and occupations kindly. So, parasitic worms long, long ago evolved a panoply of crafty evasions to our formidable defenses. This starts with, in the case of roundworms, their body cover, a tough cuticle composed of collagen and a special protein that is impervious to chemical attacks. The eggs are packaged as if to withstand a nuclear blast, with multiple resistant layers that only degrade under the right conditions, and sail through the highly acidic stomach, which dissolves most marauding bacteria. Worms' relatively large size and mobility allows them to skedaddle when they encounter some of the body's standard fortifications, such as localized inflammation and its longer-term manifestation, walling off the affected area with white blood cells. Some parasitic wrigglers opt for the wolf-in-sheep's-clothing approach, disguising themselves with coats of the host's own molecules, including antigens and a protein from blood plasma. But by far their most insidious tool is that the intruders release a plethora of substances that interfere with and sometimes control our immune response. In fact, scientists believe one type of human immune response, type 2, evolved specifically to deal with parasitic worms. Once detected, their presence sets off a number of typical reactions, including the production of immuno-globulin, high levels of certain white blood cells, and the remodeling of organs. But this full-court press does not generally save the victim, although it may help with older people who are less susceptible to heavy infestations. Meanwhile, every unwanted guest is deluging its host with body-altering substances—both secretions and excretions—that can modulate the function of white blood cells, cripple the large cells that engulf and inactivate foreign matter, and disintegrate antibodies. The net result is an age-old détente, with humans tolerating the worm infection in return for the parasites limiting themselves to inflicting survivable damages. This ancient relationship has given rise to something called the old-friends hypothesis, which reasons that humans evolved in the pres-ence of a ton of microbes—in, on, and around us—as well as parasitic worms. Because eons ago our bodies were adapted to coexist with these creatures, when they are missing—as can be the case in the Global North, our immune systems get out of whack. This is speculated to be a cause or factor in everything from asthma and gut inflammatory conditions, to autoimmune diseases—like multiple sclerosis.

When I first moved to Ecuador, an American friend invited me to an *almuerzo*, hearty lunch, in the home where he was renting a room. The meal was served in a sunny dining room overlooking a whitewashed interior patio full of potted plants and drying laundry. As I spooned up our first-course soup, I chatted with an extended family member sitting next to me, a tidily dressed, middle-aged woman who worked for the Empresa Pública Metropolitana de Agua Potable y Saneamiento de Quito, the municipal water department. I took a sip from my bottle of Güitig, Ecuador's ubiquitous spring water, and she put her hand on my arm. "Don't worry. You can drink the water here. It is perfectly potable," she said proudly. "I make sure of it." I had already been living by myself in the city for half a year, and had gradually shed many of the habits and beliefs I'd brought with me. I immediately served myself a glass from the pitcher of fresh passion fruit *licuado* in the middle of the table, made with tap water, and drank heartily. For the next three years, I fearlessly quenched my thirst from the faucet. Nothing happened, although—potty talk ahead—for the same time period, my bowel movements had the consistency of runny squash. I also ate street food prepared in giant aluminum pots and served on barely washed tin plates, ordered lettuce without fear, and made a beeline for every new tropical fruit waved at me by Ecuador's army of ambulatory vendors, part of its huge underground economy. Did I get worms? Perhaps. Did I ingest small doses of bacteria, protozoa, and viruses? Probably. But I never got sick.

For a long time, researchers have noticed that MS is much more common in Northern Europe, Canada, and the United States. For many years, it was believed that this might have to do with sun exposure and vitamin D levels, which is produced by the body in response to a type of ultraviolet light. A recent study of about two thousand cases in Germany and France supports this, correlating lower sunlight and vitamin D levels with worse disability scores. Meanwhile, scientists have come up with another theory with a strong geographic pattern: the protective effect of intestinal parasites, more frequent close to the equator. A 2006 study showed that once a threshold for human hookworm infection was met, MS prevalence drops—even in further northern and southern latitudes. The Argentinian neurologist Jorge Correale has done clinical work teasing out the possible salutary effect of having a stomach full of worms. The Fundación para la Lucha contra las Enfermedades Neurológicas de la Infancia (FLENI, Foundation to Combat Childhood Neurological Diseases), where Correale heads up the section on neuro-immunology and demyelinating diseases, has a broad practice and offers services to those of little means, who often travel hundreds of miles by public transportation to be seen. Twelve of those patients were found to have high white blood cell counts, a characteristic of worm infections. Instead of treating them, Correale searched FLENI's extensive database for twelve similar MS sufferers who did not have helminths. He then monitored both groups for four and a half years. During that period, he found that, for those with worms, the disease subsided; they had fewer flare-ups, little progression of their disabilities, and minimal new lesions on their MRIs. The presence of the parasites appeared to turn down their overactive immune systems, reducing the central nervous system inflammation that is the hallmark of the disease. The study was extended three more years, but, by year five and a half, the worm load of four of the patients began to impact their health, so they were given deworming medicine. Their symptoms promptly returned. Infecting people with "old friends" has been experimented with for celiac disease, ulcerative colitis, and Crohn's disease, as well as with MS patients in England, with some encouraging results. If the approach continues to be promising, scientists hope to isolate and synthesize some of the parasites' active molecules to cure people with pills, patches, or injections. But just as with barefoot running, any helminth-related treatments for MS and other inflammatory and autoimmune diseases should be undertaken with a recognition of their heavy toll.

∾

New parents are transfixed by their babies. So tiny! So perfect! Esmerelda, with her long limbs and solemn face, earning her the nickname *la Jueza*, the judge. Gabriela, red and swollen from her hormone-fueled, bullet-train entry to Planet Earth. Mariela, neatly folded up like a tree frog. Expressions, at first mostly accidental, pass over their features like fast-moving weather. Their mouths are seashells, wet, smooth, and precisely curved. Their arms and legs fling randomly, eliciting adorable looks of surprise by the owner. Infants watch everything, gravely, without judgment. They delight in their fingers, in their toes, in peddling their feet in the air, in being tossed, in gumming a cracker, in being cradled in your arms, in being cradled in anyone's arms. Later, they are in perpetual motion—why walk when you can run? Or climb? Or jump? So when the first injury or disorder comes, it is a shock. How could this immaculate bundle of new life be marred? But the assaults come—wounds, allergies, broken bones, learning disabilities—and accumulate.

So why does it throw us when, at some point early or late in our arc, we are diagnosed with a chronic condition or disabling disease? Even after acquiring more than a half dozen illnesses, my mother's hope never wavered. There would be a cure, and it would restore her to her flawless youthful state. The central conceit of illness—and death—is the parasite, infiltration by a malevolent, external force that, once it has gained access, controls us for its own ends. This analogy invites binarism—we will be well once we fight off the intruder, by whatever means possible: surgery, medication, visualization, apricot pit extract. At the same time, it invites passivity. If the bad thing comes from outside us, we are not responsible for the daily work of keeping it at bay, minimizing its impact once it arrives, or merely coexisting with it. Like our pre-twentieth-century notion of the earth's resources and inhabitants as boundless, this conception is archaic. After my mother died, one of her friends said to me, "Be happy she isn't suffering anymore." Our bodies are as limited as our days. Tend to them, or hasten their transformation from palace to prison.

8

The Man versus Horse Marathon

I followed Grace blindly, on one bus, then another, then another. When we got off, I was confused. It was a residential neighborhood—rows of three-deckers with pocket yards, slightly shabby, like most things in Boston were then—certainly not the place you'd find horses. We walked along the side of the road, scuffing our sneakers. It was early October, the end of a long, hot summer, and the trees, bushes, and grass looked tired.

Suddenly, Grace's golden head—she had that kind of fine hair that mats like felt—bobbed above her plaid shirt with excitement. She turned into what appeared to be a driveway leading to a ramshackle shed wedged between a house and a tiny store. Across the shed was a painted sign that read MYSTIC RIDING SCHOOL. Grace marched up to the door and flung it open.

We were brand-new friends. Each year, our elementary school broke up cliques in its class assignments, so the first weeks of September were a mad scramble. Kids sussed each other out and sized each other up. Who can I drag my desk toward so I have someone to pair up when the teacher says "find a partner"? Who will laugh uproariously when I fake vomit on my cafeteria sloppy Joe? Who will be the best ally for recess capture the flag? And, if the school hours went without a hiccup, who will I hang out with afterward?

But the reason Grace and I ended up with each other was because we were both quiet.

My quiet was the kind that came from liking books and drawing and knowing enough to keep my head down in a struggling public school. Grace's, from the fact that her parents had recently divorced, her mother was working a minimum-wage job, and she went home every day to an empty apartment. (This being the 1970s, I was the odd one out because my parents were still married and my mother was a housewife.) Grace covered it up with a cool-kid exterior, but I could sense that deep inside, she was sad and scared. Maybe that's why, within a few weeks of beginning sixth grade, she invited me, someone she hardly knew, to share her most sacred activity: riding.

Inside the stables, an older Black man looked up from something he was repairing and smiled.

"Come to give D'Artagnan his exercise?" he asked. Grace nodded.

"And I brought my friend. She's never ridden before." Embarrassing, but at least having my inexperience out in the open meant the owner might have pity when he matched me with one of his herd. Grace immediately plunged deeper into the stable, chattering away in a mostly foreign language: tacks and bridles, reins and stirrups, blankets and bits. After about five minutes, she emerged guiding the tallest horse I'd ever seen—silver white, with a cream mane, and a tense, erect bearing. I shrank. They expected me to climb on this monster? Grace handed me the reins.

"Here."

Then she returned to where, in another stall, Charlie Jordan was preparing a short and stocky brown mare. Grace led her to the stable door, and again handed me the reins.

"This is Miss Molly. She's a little lazy, so you have to kick her hard. But she'll be just right for you." I breathed a sigh of relief as she took the reins to the giant.

"My horse's name is D'Artagnan," Grace said slowly, drawing her hand lovingly down the horse's muscular neck. "When I grow up," she said, "I'm going to buy him."

Getting on Miss Molly wasn't as hard as I feared. Charlie Jordan interlocked his two hands and held them out for me to step in. Once I did, he lifted me onto the saddle. Miss Molly's ears twitched. Somehow, it didn't feel like a friendly acknowledgment of my presence.

Grace didn't need any help. She inserted her left foot into the stirrup and swung her right leg in a perfect arc around the horse's powerful flanks. Then she settled back into the saddle beaming. In school, Grace almost disappeared, but up there, astride D'Artagnan, she was a different person.

My relationship with Miss Molly was troubled from the start. Grace, sitting ramrod straight, gently dug her heels in D'Artagnan's sides, and he started walking. I did the same, and nothing happened. I kicked. I kicked again, harder. Miss Molly turned and gave me a look that said, "What the hell are you doing?" I'm pretty sure she wouldn't have left the stable except that the owner gave her a swat on her flanks with a switch.

"Manners, young lady!" he grumbled. Miss Molly lurched forward with the equine equivalent of a shrug and an exaggerated eye roll.

"Hold the reins firmly," Jordan said. "Pull gently in the direction you want to go." I tried, but honestly, it was Miss Molly's show from the beginning. Luckily, she seemed to have a bit of a thing for D'Artagnan. We clopped over the asphalt and caught up with them when they halted to enter the traffic circle.

"Ready?" said Grace. In that moment she glowed like one of the heroines—the plucky kind that save their families' lives, not the passive princesses—in the fairy stories I devoured as a young child.

Quite a few cars went by before one stopped to let our horses amble the half circle of the rotary. They had obviously done this before—they headed straight for a narrow dirt track weaving into the high, yellow grass. The open area was sandwiched between the river, edged by a few tall trees, and the parkway, where cars whizzed to and fro.

"Okay," Grace said. "Now we're going to trot." I tried not to look terrified. So far, we had probably covered all of one hundred yards, walking. "Don't freak out. All you have to do is hold on. Just grab the horn." It was a Western-style saddle, probably safer with the newbies. "Hold on with your thighs, and relax."

D'Artagnan set off; he seemed to be picking up each foot and setting it down precisely. Grace, although her back was straighter than ever, seemed to be moving with him from the waist down. It looked good. I kicked Miss Molly. Nothing. I kicked her again. This time she turned and shot me that look—only this time I took it to mean, "Now that it's just you and me, not on your life, sweetheart."

"What are you waiting for?" Grace called from the other end of the grassy area.

"She won't move," I said. Grace turned D'Artagnan, trotted back, and reached over and slapped Miss Molly on the rump. The mare snorted and set off in a tortuous up-and-down motion. Was this what an earthquake felt like—the ground beneath you suddenly unreliable? I clapped my hands on the horn and managed to hold on all the way across the field. We practiced trotting a bit more, and then Grace declared we were ready to canter.

"It's so fun! You're going to love it!" Again, she told me to hold the horn and sit back. Then she dug her heels into D'Artagnan. I watched them take off across the grass. The horse's hindquarters contracted and stretched rhythmically under his body, like a giant loping rabbit. Grace jostled along. They accelerated, turned at the woods, and came back.

"Your turn!"

"I don't think so. I'm just a beginner."

"It's easy," she said, reaching over and giving Miss Molly a huge whack. The mare whinnied, then started undulating the same way

D'Artagnan had. As the grass sped by, I noted white and purple asters peeking between feathery spikes. The sky was blue and dotted with fluffy clouds. Before I knew it, we were at the other side. I felt as though I'd been flying.

Grace cantered over, and then we both cantered back. And back again. D'Artagnan and Miss Molly started having good-natured races. I think Miss Molly was trying to show off by keeping up with him. D'Artagnan, true to his noble stature, restrained himself so that the difference in their abilities wasn't comical. I could have kept cantering all afternoon, but suddenly Grace got bored.

"Let's go on a trail ride," she said.

"It's getting late." I didn't know what time it was, but with the bus rides and all, I expected it was at least 4:30 P.M., and I knew my mother would worry if I hadn't shown up by 5:00 P.M. on a school day.

"Come on," Grace said. "Don't be a party pooper." She turned the reins toward the trail, pressed her heels into D'Artagnan's side, and headed off to the other side, where the grass gave way to trees—maples, oaks, and sumac. Miss Molly, warmed up by all the cantering, followed of her own accord. Each time the horses' hooves struck the path, a small cloud of dust rose up. I felt the sun slanting, the afternoon cooling, and suddenly, longed to be home, sitting at the kitchen counter, while my mother busied herself with dinner. Up ahead, the path dipped into darkness—the woods that unfurled against the river banks. I watched Grace's back; it hadn't seemed to bend the entire time we'd been riding.

Then she disappeared. D'Artagnan's glistening flanks, which had framed her like the two sides of a heart, were also gone. He had stumbled. Grace had flown over his head and was facedown in the underbrush. Miss Molly stood stock still. My mind raced. What should I do? Jump off my horse and run to Grace? Grab D'Artagnan's reins?—he was already starting to raise himself from the uneven ground. Tie both horses to trees and run to the highway to wave frantically, in hopes that an adult would stop and help me? I was terrified. But whatever I did, the first step would have to be dismount. I leaned forward over the horn, clutching it under me. I disengaged my right foot and worked it over the mare's broad back. Once I got it to the other side, I'd dangle my legs as far as I could and then let go.

Just then, Grace pushed herself back into a kneeling position, wiped the debris off her scratched and bleeding face and torso, and clambered to her feet.

"Don't think you're going anywhere, wise guy," she said, grabbing D'Artagnan's hanging reins. She looked at me and Miss Molly, still probably fifty feet away. "That was a bad one." She didn't seem to be perturbed, just pulled D'Artagnan over to an open area, and hopped back up. I still hadn't spoken. My mind was coursing: fear and wonder, surprise and relief. How come she wasn't crying? How could she get back on the horse? How could she be nosing D'Artagnan back toward the woods as if nothing had happened? What made Grace so fearless? I couldn't imagine, but I wanted to be that way, too.

We finished up our trail ride and brought the horses back to the stable, unfolding the $10 bills we'd stuffed deep into our pockets for Jordan.

"D'Artagnan threw me again," Grace commented.

"Got to be careful of that one," the owner said.

"Not his fault. A root," Grace said.

When I got home, it was dark and close to 7:00 P.M. My mother asked me where I'd been. "With Grace, that friend from school," I said. She hmmed distractedly and handed me my plate.

∽

It begins with a shout. "'Have a good time out there!' And you're like, is that even the start of the race?" says Nick Coury, an ultramarathoner, who glows even through Zoom, a quality that seems half extraordinary health and half laser-focused intensity. "And then the horses take off and leave you in a cloud of dust." He's talking about the Man Against Horse Race, a Prescott, Arizona, tradition since 1983, the result of a bar bet between county supervisor and runner L. Gheral Brownlow and officer with the city's police department and cowboy Steve Rafters. There are three distances: the twelve-mile "fun run" for those testing the waters; the twenty-five miler for the multitudes, still stuck in the marathon mindset; and the real deal, the one that gives humans a fighting chance against nature's best long-distance runners, a fifty-mile trek over Mingus Mountain. The races all begin—with slightly staggered times—in the same place, the wide-open plains of the Fain Cattle Ranch in the Black Hills Mountain range of central Arizona, already at about five thousand feet above sea level and accounting for its mild year-round climate. "Yeah," says race organizer Ron Barrett, both an ultramarathoner and an endurance rider himself. "It all starts out pretty wild. I mean, the runners, they want to get out right away, you know, and the start of the race goes through a big wash. It's kind of tricky. So I always tell everybody, just take it easy . . . the horse has to let the runners get out first, and then it opens up, and they take off."

I've contacted Coury because he's done the unthinkable: outrun the fastest horse, not only once, but twice. (There have been previous races where runners crossed the finish line first, but since horses must stop for a total of an hour and fifteen minutes, a period subtracted from their overall ride time, no person had won the race outright.) Humans have also occasionally triumphed in the well-known Man versus Horse Marathon in Llanwrtyd Wells, Wales, a mere twenty-two miles long, as well as in the two other such events—one in Dores, Scotland, the other in Central North Island, New Zealand. "You think that there's no way a man could ever beat a horse," Coury says. "But one of the reasons that we can is that humans have a lot of physiological adaptations that are very good for long-distance running." Sure. We've got long legs, fixed heads, muscular buttocks, sweat glands all over our bodies, and minimal body hair, but none of these things explain how Coury did what thousands of other runners tried and failed to.

After about five miles of rolling hills, the Man Against Horse course gets serious. Grassy chaparral gives way to pinon and juniper, and the trail cuts back and forth through a canyon, Grapevine Gulch. At mile sixteen, the route reaches a ridge with panoramic views of the Verde Valley below and the first mandatory, half-hour veterinary stop. "The pulse [of the horses] has to come down," Barrett says. "And then the veterinarian will check the heart rate, the capillary refill, how hydrated they are, how their gut sounds, and then they have to trot out and trot back and make sure they're sound. So they're not lame and limping. And if they don't meet all of that criteria, especially the soundness, then they get pulled. They're out of the race." The horses are given water and feed, often supplemented with electrolyte powders with names like Summer Games, Rein Water, Apple-a-Day, and Endura-Max, and cooled by sponging them with water. (Veterinary checks and holds are part of the rules of the American Endurance Ride Conference.) It was shortly after this first vet check and emerging into a stand of ponderosa pines, that Coury realized something was different about the 2019 race, his third.

"I know some of the riders, like Troy [Eckard] and I know he's one of the top performers—he's won the race before. So I knew if someone was going to be there, it would probably be him. He was way ahead of the rest of the horses. . . . And so when I passed him [at the vet check], I knew where I should get caught. . . . I'd never been ahead at that point." Coury began barreling across the ridge, which offers several flats—perfect spots for a galloping horse to overtake him, but no horse appeared. Then the route doubled down, wending its way northeast and up, and Coury stopped thinking about anything else but just getting through it. "The backside of the course is like a really steep climb," he says. "I think it's 1,500 feet in two miles. [It's 1,800 in three, according to Barrett] . . . And it tends to be rocky, kind of slippery with loose dirt. It gets really narrow where there's bushes growing from both sides, and there's big boulders in the way that you have to climb over. . . . It gets exhausting for me. And so I have to imagine [that for] a horse with different biomechanics, some of those parts have to be even harder." Finally, Coury summited, thirty-three miles into the race, and passed the second vet stop, this one with a hold time of forty-five minutes. There were definitely no equine contenders in front of him.

I'm impressed by the level of concern for the animals, but baffled about why there isn't the equivalent for the human participants. "The funniest part of it is that we have to stop these horses, and we look at them and make sure everything's okay," chuckles Matthew Houser, lead veterinarian for the event for over twenty-five years. "But those runners just keep going!" It's not like they don't take care of business on the trail. There are aid stations approximately every five miles, stocked with bottled water, snacks, first aid kits, friendly volunteers, and, sporadically, portable toilets. But whether they stop once, a few times, constantly, or not at all is left up to the discretion of the athletes. I ask Barrett why. He shrugs. "If they're not feeling well, or for whatever reason, like I said, dehydration, cramping, upset stomach, all those things occur anyways, with most runners doing fifty- and hundred-mile runs. But a lot of times, guys that are experienced runners, they work through that stuff. You know, they take salt tablets, and there's so many supplements out there today to help you get through an event."

By contrast, overriding a horse can so interfere with its basic functions that it can quickly spiral into organ damage or worse. In 2018 Barack Obama, a New Zealand horse in a 120-kilometer endurance race in South Carolina, had to be euthanized for kidney issues after running the first loop. That race, held in hot and humid September, was ultimately canceled after an unusually high number of horses—53 of 120—showed signs of metabolic distress. "It was unprecedented. Never happened before," says David Marlin, an internationally renowned expert on equine thermoregulation who was there serving as a climate mitigation specialist for Fédération Equestre Internationale (FEI), the world governing body for equestrian sports. "And so a meeting was called, and it was decided to hold the event, cancel, abandon whatever you want to use, on horse welfare grounds." Intense exertion, especially in the heat, can lead them to "develop severe electrolyte imbalances that lead to abnormal heart function," he explains. But there are several other factors that make this situation much more dangerous for horses than for human beings. The animals have voluntary control over their blood flow, at least for short periods. "I'm going to direct more of the blood flow that I've got to more of my cardiac output, to the muscle, and I'm going to compromise my thermoregulation. So my temperature was going up like this"—his fingers spike up—"but I'm running faster." The other point Marlin makes is the additional burden of the rider on the horse's cooling—since no heat can escape from under the saddle—and load. "To make [the Man Against Horse Race] a fair race, the runners should really have a rucksack on their backs carrying 17 percent of their body weight."

Horses and humans are the champion long-distance runners of the animal kingdom. We are also the champion sweaters, dripping profusely all over our bodies during exertion and hot conditions. These two things are not unrelated. Other mammals may perspire a bit, but most rely on panting; wallowing; having big, capillary-rich ears; or lounging in the shade to dissipate excess heat. But people have one additional adaptation, one that guarantees our supremacy over ponies in the thermoregulatory department. There are two basic kinds of sweat glands. Apocrine secrete an oily fluid containing proteins, hormones, and lipids; most animals, including horses, have these all over their bodies. During activity, horses may lose ten to fifteen liters of apocrine gland sweat. But because it is rich in the aforementioned substances, plus one unique to the species, latherin (which causes a foamy appearance and wets their coats for improved evaporation and cooling), horses' sweat is hypertonic—it has more electrolytes than their blood and other cells. Covering long distances, especially in warm weather, depletes these, causing problems with muscle function, blood pressure, and heart rhythm—and can even lead to death. Unlike the rest of our mammalian brethren, humans only have apocrine glands in our stinky spots. On the other hand, we have two to four million eccrine sweat glands all over our bodies, while animals, including horses, only have a few of these and only on their feet. The composition of eccrine gland sweat is mostly water with a tiny bit of salt. It is hypotonic, which means it has a lower electrolyte content than that of the body. This means that, while endurance athletes can lose from two thirds to two liters of fluid an hour, according to a 2019 study by the Gatorade Sports Science Institute, as long as they stay hydrated, they can run for about five hours straight. And then, they only need a bit of salt—easily replaced with a tablet, or better yet, a snack such as olives, pretzels, or a cheese cube—to continue without any ill effects.

By now, the sun is high in the sky, the tree cover is sparse, and the temperature is close to 80 degrees Fahrenheit. Coury, who is from Scottsdale, Arizona, works out in the heat and considers his capacity to contend with these conditions a tactical advantage. "Most of my trainings are in the morning just for scheduling, but I actually try to do some runs in the really bad heat. So, like, in the summer, I'll do some runs when it's 105 degrees, 110 degrees. Well, not very many because you have to be realistic! With that heat, I have found that the physiological adaptations are really nice—after the fact—it's not nice during! But once I get used to it, my body adapts, and then I go anywhere cooler, it's like Superman coming from Krypton to earth, and he breathes this easier atmosphere and has superpowers." Horses can be heat acclimated as well; however, their less reliable cooling system means that owners must always be wary. "With a horse and a rider, it's more difficult to get through the course than a runner," Barrett says. "Because you not only have to take care of yourself as a rider, you also have to know your horse and what he is capable of doing on a given day, with the terrain, with the heat, with the elevation, the climb, and the speed you're going." I am astounded that someone would not only risk their animal companion, but a major investment—a horse can cost anywhere from the price of decent used car to a Lamborghini. Marianne Ironside, founder of the horse welfare group Clean Endurance International, explains it this way: "Endurance riders tend to be quite stubborn, because we have to ride a long time. And we have to ride through pain barriers and fatigue barriers. And when you've worked so hard, and you're halfway through the ride, you're absolutely determined that you're going to finish it. It's very tempting to push your horse that little bit further than you really should be pushing it."

The mountaintop, at 7,818 feet, is a revelation. From here, you have a stunning view of the Verde Valley, the red rocks of Sedona, Humphreys Peak, and the two-hundred-mile-long Mogollon Rim. Then comes the descent, by turns gradual and punishing. In the easy parts, there are pines, needles underfoot, and filtered sunlight. You float. In the difficult ones, there are ruts and rocks and steep drops. Your quads brace against the impact and your joints fight gravity. But after a while, Coury realizes he's on the home stretch. He passes the final vet area, a "stop and go," where there's no hold, just a quick check to make sure the horses' hearts are sixty-four beats or under per minute and that they aren't lame. "It's like an unbelievable feeling, the last ten miles leading up to the finish. I'm like paranoid that I'm going to get caught, but at the same time, I know ten miles from the finish is doable. Both [of the previous] years, I had run it well enough that I know I have something left, I'm not fading, I'm not dying. I think I can start pushing. So I actually just started picking up progressively more and more. And, you know, every time I pick it up a little more, like you get more adrenaline pumping, and you're like, 'Okay, I'm still not fading, I'm gonna push a little harder.' And then, 'I think I've got this.' I push a little harder. And so it's like this crescendo all the way until the finish. And by the time I'm getting to the finish, I'm just sprinting as hard as I can, basically. And then you cross that line after being out there all day. And it's just like this overwhelming rush of emotions all coming in. 'I did it. And I can stop now. And I can't believe I did it.' It's just these overwhelming feelings of ecstasy." Coury had completed the fifty-mile course in six hours, fourteen minutes, and twenty-four seconds. He knew he was the first runner to cross the finish line—a feat that, while not frequent, had happened a few times before. But win the race overall? He could only hope. And wait. When the first horse finally got there, Crixius, ridden by Tammy Gagnon, a full two and a half additional hours had passed. Coury was not only the first runner to cross the finish line, his run time had surpassed that of the first horse's by an hour and fifteen minutes. He was now officially the first person to ever beat a horse in the race. (Although to be fair, Gagnon says she was just there for fun, so when frontrunner Eckard's horse stumbled, she was unprepared to make up for her leisurely pace earlier in the race. In 2018 Eckard had won the race outright, with a time of six hours and forty-six minutes.) "He blew me away," Houser says of Coury. "And my wife. She couldn't believe this guy. Because he's running the race and cutting off enough time that he could have stopped with the horses for the half hour, forty-five minutes, and five minutes, and he still would have beat them. Fast. I'd never seen anybody that could run like that. And he always looks really good at the end, too. Yeah. So yeah. As far as truly beating the horse, he's the only one I know."

But Coury's remarkable victory jogs something in Houser's memory and he begins to tell me about the runner who, in all these decades, most impressed him. It's as if he had been sent to tactfully guide me to American distance running's Indigenous origins. "And then we had an Indian guy that came in and he always amazed me because he'd come running through and he would almost beat [the horses] with the stops. But the amazing thing to me was when you get to the bottom, you know, most of these guys are barely walking, and after running fifty miles, he'd be down there playing football with the kids. Or one time he asked if he could have his medal early because he was going to an all-night dance on the reservation. I always liked that guy. Very quiet. But man could he run—and he just looked like he hadn't done anything. One night I sat with his parents at the dinner. And they said, 'Yeah, one morning he got up and just took off running. Then later that night, we got a phone call. And he wanted us to come pick him up. And so we asked him where he was.' They said he had run 130 miles. He was an amazing guy. And unfortunately, he was running down in Phoenix, I believe, and was hit by a car."

"For me, what I will remember most about Dennis, or Danny as his family calls him, is his tremendous inner strength. While there was never any doubt as to his physical strength, which was made clear to me every time he powered ahead of me on a hot, desert mountain, it was his spiritual strength—his inner centeredness—that made a lasting impression on me and which I will never forget," writes his occasional running buddy Andy Jones-Wilkins in a blog post after his death in June 2015. On the trail and off, Dennis Poolheco was humble and community-minded—during a race, he thought nothing of circling back to support a struggling fellow runner. His calm and generosity belied a difficult past. His mother had passed away shortly after he was born, and he'd been raised by his paternal grandparents—David, a runner, and Evelyn, a potter, in Tewa, a village in the Hopi Tribe's First Mesa reservation. During his teenage years, he moved to Winslow, Arizona, a town about seventy miles away. Although Poolheco did well in high school, graduating in the top ten, according to his uncle Walter Poolheco, as a young man, he became addicted to alcohol, losing most of his twenties and thirties to the disease. When he finally decided to quit, with the help of a longtime friend, "he started running to keep himself away from that," says his ex-wife.

In no time at all, Poolheco became a local legend, entering and winning ultramarathons, including coming in first among the runners four
consecutive years (and second in 2005, his final year) at the Man Against
Horse Race. He also used his running as a force for good, encouraging
Hopi youth to do the sport, creating a running group for Hopis practicing
sobriety, and honoring elders and his community by tying together mean-
ingful places—for example, his mother's birth village, his grandparents'
village, and the town he grew up in—with distance runs. "There's a lot
of time out there to think. I think about people who are sick or having
problems and say prayers for them while I run," Poolheco once said. In
this, he was continuing a tradition handed down through generations.
"You see throughout history that the Hopi are running for various
reasons, for different purposes," explains Matthew Sakiestewa Gilbert,
head of the Department of American Indian Studies at the University
of Arizona, a Hopi Tribe member, and author of *Hopi Runners: Crossing
the Terrain between Indian and American*. "There's always this concept
that wherever they are running on the earth, wherever they are running
beyond the mesa, beyond the Hopi mesas and their ancestral homelands,
they are running for their people, they're keeping their families in
mind, they're keeping their village in mind."

One of the ways that Hopi athletes train is to look to the animal
world for inspiration—and to emulate them. "Wild animals are very
graceful runners, depending on the animal. They're beautiful runners,
beautiful runners. If you study a deer or antelope, how it runs so efficiently, so gracefully, you will learn to 'dance on the earth,'" Gilbert says.
Of course, one of the most elegant runners on the planet is the horse,
which, while it may or may not have inhabited the continent at the same
time as Indigenous peoples, originated in North America. A dog-sized
tropical mammal with spread-out toes, it appeared after an asteroid hit
earth sixty-six million years ago, blanketing the atmosphere with a layer
of dust and debris that halted plant photosynthesis and extinguished

three quarters of all flora and fauna species. In the new, drier world that emerged, the horses' ancestors thrived on grassy plains. By 12,000 B.C.E., some had migrated north to Asia; those that remained went extinct. But since humans are estimated to have arrived to the Americas from Asia about 20,000 B.C.E.—crossing the Bering Strait, which was not then covered by the sea, and are definitely present by 16,000 B.C.E., there are 8,000–4,000 years of likely coexistence. Then, the horse disappears from the continent, only to return, after a circuitous journey across the Eurasian Steppe and a new relationship with humans, first as a foodstuff, and then as a cutting-edge military technology, with Spanish and French colonists. A few escaped or were abandoned and populated the plains with herds of wild horses, many of which remain to this day. Although most scholars agree that, at least by the arrival of Europeans, there were no native horses in the Americas, one Indigenous researcher, Yvette Running Horse Collin, disputes this narrative, claiming some breeds survived—seven different nations have origin stories attributing the animal to a gift from the Creator, she says—and has started a sanctuary for their preservation.

∽

The maple and oak woods, laced with ferns, gave way to a little rise that opened onto a hill, green with July grass. Meadowdale Stables in Guilford, Vermont, was a few miles from the low mountain where my great-grandmother had lived and died and where my grandmother was born. The terrain—gentle and intricate—was imprinted on me in babyhood and inhabits my dreams. The house, unpainted gray, dilapidated, with a ladder against one wall and a woodbox to the side of the door, was from the New England of my earliest memories, poor and plain.

I pulled into the gravel driveway and parked opposite the house, and my sister did the same. Mariela and her slightly younger cousin, Aviva, tumbled out of the backseats and went running toward the red barn, which, unlike the house, was well kept-up.

"Horses!" they exclaimed. They were far older than I was when I first went riding with Grace, but close to the age when, for two years, a couple friends and I took riding lessons (the period ended when one of the group broke her collarbone). On Saturdays, we trekked—via bus, subway, another bus, and then a mile's walk—to a suburban stable. In an outdoor ring at the top of a hill, we learned to sit in a saddle, post, trot, gallop, and jump. Afterward, I was elated. Five feet off the ground, leaning into my sit bones, my thighs lightly squeezed, I was always—with good reason—slightly scared. But I was also learning how to talk and listen to a powerful and majestic animal, a skill that connected me to millennia of human history—and to the strong person I longed to be. Now, for her fourteenth birthday, I wanted to share that feeling with Mariela and her cousin.

It took us a while to locate the owner, Elsie Starr, who was as rugged and weather-beaten as her house. I guessed she was close to eighty. "Go to the barn. Jessica will take care of the paperwork and saddle up some horses for you. But before that, we'll have you groom the horses. So you get to know them. And they get to know you." The paperwork was a liability form in which I assumed responsibility for all risks and waived my right to sue for any untoward events related to our visit. There was also a bolded advisory: WARNING UNDER VERMONT LAW, AN EQUINE ACTIVITY SPONSOR IS NOT LIABLE FOR ANY INJURY TO, OR DEATH OF, A PARTICIPANT IN EQUINE ACTIVITIES RESULTING FROM THE INHERENT RISK OF EQUINE ACTIVITIES THAT ARE OBVIOUS AND NECESSARY PURSUANT TO 12 V.S.A. §1039. From a nearby paddock, Jessica Poole collected Merwin, a big pinto with a splotchy brown and white coat.

"Here," she said. "You're the experienced rider. He's a sweetheart. Very intelligent and responsive." I led Merwin to the barn, tied his reins to a post, and brushed him, leaning into his shoulder, talking to him in a low voice. I was so eager, it was hard for me to tear myself away from him to check in on the others. Mariela was fine, but Aviva had been given a pony that, perhaps sensing her uncertainty, was turning to give her the stink eye every time she laid the curry comb on his side.

Once in the indoor ring, Starr stopped her horse in the middle and began shouting out instructions while Poole led our string of horses back and forth. Their approach, called centered riding, is like equine medita-tion. We were instructed to breathe deeply, feel gravity's pull, move slowly and deliberately, and to drop the reins—even rank beginners. Which, of course, was a stunt designed to show us that the seat is where horse and rider are one. After mastering the basics, Starr asked, "Do you want to go for a short trail ride?" Of course we did.

She led us across the street at the horse crossing sign and up a rough embankment. As her voice faded into the distance, I savored the dappled sunlight, the happy exclamations of my daughter and her cousin, and the feeling of peace that crept over me, and concentrated on keeping my weight evenly distributed on Merwin's back as his hooves slipped in the rutted earth. I wasn't frightened, but sitting there, at the same height as the branches hanging over the trail, I knew he could stumble, that I could fall, that he could fall, that this activity, so transcendent, was, by its nature, dangerous, and that those two things were bound together.

The end of our lesson abruptly returned me to the more usual sham-bolic course of my life. I'd neglected to follow the instructions on the website and in the email correspondence to arrange our session that all payments were to be in cash. I sheepishly took out my credit card. "You can't? Don't worry, I'll just go to an ATM." I felt terrible; was she anticipating my $160 to pay for groceries or some other necessities? Two hours later, I called Starr from a gas station, where I'd stopped to fill my empty tank. "So, so sorry. I tried to take a shortcut and got lost on the dirt roads in the woods. We almost ran out of gas, and it would take me another half hour to get back there, and it's late, and the kids are tired.

Can I mail you a check?" In her thank-you note when she received it, Starr said she hoped we'd come back. Two years later, with COVID-19 raging in the fall of 2020, we did. Just like before, the girls burst out of the cars once we'd arrived. Starr opened the door to her house in greeting, then walked to join us, painfully dragging her left leg behind her.

"Casey will be leading you in your lesson today," she said, without a flicker of self-pity. "Took a fall a while back and my leg shattered. Broke in eight places, and it just didn't set right."

~

There comes a point in every summer, usually between mid-July and mid-August, when I start to wonder if I'm dying. Could I have some undiagnosed (additional) disease, like my friend's sister-in-law who passed the same week her Christmas Day fatigue so alarmed her family that they took her to the emergency room, where they found she was riddled with cancer? I am heavy, exhausted, slow. My runs, always later in the morning sun than I wish (living among night owls means that the house doesn't usually quiet till after 1:00 A.M.), feel like treks through quicksand. I pour sweat, losing a couple pounds in the hour I am out, and constantly mop my brow with a handkerchief I tie around my wrist to keep sunscreen from getting in my eyes. In my basement office, the atmosphere is thick and my brain throbs, as if I were nursing a constant hangover. In the afternoon, despite my three cups of coffee and mug of tea, I may wander upstairs and stretch out under the ceiling fan in our bedroom. I shut my eyes for a second and wake up forty minutes later. Summer in Boston is a steam bath. In fact, the average July day, with a temperature of 92 degrees Fahrenheit and a relative humidity of 55 percent feels the same as a blazing hot Arizona day of 105 degrees Fahrenheit and a relative humidity of 31 percent—take that, Nick Coury! Both result in a wet-bulb globe temperature (WBGT—literally the temperature taken when the bulb is wrapped in wet cloth and placed in direct sunlight, showing how much heat can be evaporated for cooling) of about 79 degrees Fahrenheit, which, while not dangerous, is close. At 82 degrees Fahrenheit WBGT, football coaches start watching their at-risk players carefully and are advised to provide at least three rest breaks per hour. At 92 degrees Fahrenheit WBGT, practice is canceled. (And above 95 Fahrenheit WBGT is uninhabitable, a serious problem for those in the southern Persian Gulf and northern South Asia, according to a 2020 study done at the California Institute of Technology and Columbia University.) This explains a lot. On a hot day here, say 95 degrees Fahrenheit, with a typical relative humidity of 65 percent, we Bostonians are close to the red danger zone for being active outside, with a real feel of 114–121 degrees Fahrenheit, according to the National Weather Service Heat Index Chart. No wonder my July and August slogs through the streets feel like marathons.

Anne von Rosen hadn't planned on becoming a jockey. Born in central Germany to an outdoorsy family, her homeopathic physician father introduced her to riding at a young age and got her her own Icelandic pony when she was nine. As a young woman, she worked on a breeding farm and then landed a job cleaning the stalls and exercising the horses at various European racetracks. Thinking she might enter the veterinary field, in 1998, she became an assistant at the Hagyard Equine Medical Institute in Lexington, Kentucky, but soon discovered she "missed galloping too much," she says in an interview with the website Female Jockeys. She then found a position as an assistant trainer at the William Harrigan breaking and horse training farm, Miacomet, also in Kentucky, then as a trainer in Pierre, South Dakota. She ran her first race as a jockey in Tampa, Florida, in 2001, the first of over four thousand, of which she won more than six hundred.

Then, at the end of a March 2014 race at Turf Paradise in Phoenix, in which she placed second, "I remember galloping out thinking the mare had run a huge race. The next thing I know, I'm lying on the ground," von Rosen said to the *Paulick Report*, a horse racing news source. "I couldn't feel my legs, but the strange thing was it wasn't scary. I knew what had happened, and I accepted it. I always have. I think people don't know how dangerous this sport is." Von Rosen's horse had fallen, landing on top of her, completely severing her spine at the fifth thoracic vertebra, about shoulder-blade level. She was rushed to the hospital, where she had a seven-hour operation and then another one a couple days later. In an instant, her life had changed. But she hadn't lost the fearlessness and tenacity that had brought her success as a jockey. She would now apply it to regaining as much mobility as she could. In this journey, she has been supported by the Permanently Disabled Jockeys Fund, which provides financial and other assistance to sixty jockeys who've suffered catastrophic spinal cord and brain injuries. (Serious injury rates are high for anyone involved in equestrian sports, affecting some 20 percent of all riders, professional and recreational.)

It's been a long road. When I spoke with von Rosen, she was standing, using a brace. I noticed that her neck and arms were slender and well-muscled; somehow, despite the fact that she could not use her legs, she was keeping, not only fit, but, it appeared, in top condition. I asked her to describe a typical day. "My life is not very exciting," she apologizes. She explains that everything takes a very long time: getting dressed, preparing and eating meals, and cleaning up. Then she does training and exercising using equipment she has at home. "Pretty much all I do is work on myself to get better, you know?" I ask her if she is still expecting to recover some function, and she tells me: "Everything!" I am momentarily dumbstruck, then I ask how much progress she's made. "I can ride a horse and trot a little bit. I'm not galloping yet. Not quite. I can stand. I can walk a little bit. Not very good. But I can take some steps." In fact, she is learning para reining, which allows people of varying physical abilities to participate in reining, a western US tradition that showcases the control a rider has over the horse and has been described as the equestrian version of figure skating. For now, her riding is limited to one or two half-hour sessions a week, but as von Rosen gains trunk stability, she hopes to increase it. "The horses give me my legs back. And it's something I can do. Not as good, but at least I can still do it. And it's just a sense of freedom."

Not being able to walk, reduced independence, and the time investment for the simplest tasks are only the most obvious outcomes of an accident like von Rosen's. There are many other bodily impacts, from having to get up in the middle of the night to empty a catheter bag, maintaining a bowel schedule, visually inspecting her own limbs for cuts that could get infected, having difficulty coughing, tiring faster, and not being able to regulate body heat below her injury. That means that, for the first few years anyway, she couldn't sweat, putting her at risk of overheating on a hot day or during exertion. Similarly, her body didn't convey the signal to constrict blood vessels to reduce heat loss in lower temperatures, which means that von Rosen also got cold easily, often piling on the clothes even though she lives in Phoenix. Things have improved with all the rehab work she's done. Some of her sweat function has returned, and now she warms up quicker when it's chilly. One of the many organizations that has offered much needed financial assistance to help von Rosen stay active is Will2Walk, which, according to its website description, "provides funding for equipment or services to support your passion for a healthy, active and independent lifestyle." In 2018 the nonprofit gave von Rosen money to pay for strength-training therapy.

Will2Walk is the brainchild of Rich Hamill, who also lives with a spinal cord injury. On a February day in 1992, with temperatures hovering just above freezing, Hamill and his best friend Chuck set out on a ski trip feeling on top of the world: they'd helped power the Deckerville High School football team to victory dozens of times; they would graduate in a few months, with the ceremonies and celebrations that entails; and they were about to head off to college. Then the car hit black ice and Chuck, who was at the wheel, couldn't keep it from hitting a tree. When Hamill came to, he was in the hospital and paralyzed. His injury was at the base of the neck, at the sixth and seventh cervical vertebrae; this left him with some movement in his arms and hands, but none in his trunk or legs. Good-bye, plans. For the next year and a half, he just did physical therapy. He had to relearn all the fine motor skills, including writing, using workarounds for dysfunctional muscles, and, with an adapted vehicle, regained some autonomy. While still living with his parents, he drove himself to Saint Claire Community College, forty-one miles away, majoring in management. "It took me a little longer than I had planned. . . . And after I graduated, I worked in Michigan for a year, saved my money, and moved out to Arizona with $1,000 in my pocket, having no idea what I was gonna do."

What he did, after a year-and-a-half search in which he faced, for the first time, discrimination for being disabled, was find a job in the insurance industry. He also returned to sports. "When I first got paralyzed, I knew a couple of guys that were in wheelchairs and had spinal cord injuries, but everybody I spent time with was able-bodied. . . . When I moved to Arizona, I was pretty much on my own. So I was out doing things and I found the Arizona Disabled Sports, which was in Mesa, Arizona, and I went and attended a rugby meet. And I met a bunch of other people with spinal cord injuries and who had different disabilities. And it gave me a real chance to get a true picture of life [when you are disabled]. For others, not just myself. So I got involved with that community pretty early on."

Will2Walk came out of Hamill's appreciation for the fact that he was injured in Michigan, which, until the law changed in 2020, mandated no-fault insurance policies for all vehicles, covering bodily injury costs for life. In Arizona, and through a motivational speaking gig, which flew him around the country, he spoke with many other people living with spinal cord injuries. Their recoveries, independence, and capacity to live life to the fullest were hampered by their inability to purchase equipment, adaptations, and training. "For my situation, a new wheelchair or modifications to the home, or adaptation to the vehicle, yeah, my insurance covers all that until I die. And I didn't realize what a big deal that was until I met others that didn't have that, and how much money everything costs. Realizing how lucky I was, I'm like, you know, how do I help the spinal cord community?" Hamill, who, to keep in shape, was hand-cycling thirty to forty miles a day, decided to raise funds by hand-cycling across the country. Then he tore his shoulder. Temporarily laid up, he sent solicitations to everyone he knew and finally scraped together the first $25,000 for the nonprofit, telling people that "my goal is to help every person with a spinal cord injury in the country that needs help. If it's financial aid, for education, if it's medical supplies, if it's modifications, [as long as] it's anything to keep them healthy, active, and moving in life. . . . And I was overwhelmed with the response. And that has motivated me to keep going harder."

To date, Will2Walk has provided over $270,000 to more than one hundred people living with life-changing traumatic injuries. They do not yet have a full-fledged mentoring program, although Hamill hopes to someday. In the meantime, he has personally mentored over forty-five people in figuring out how to be physically active. "If you're like me, for example, I don't have any grip. I can type, I have decent fine motor skills and little things, but I can't hold a weight. I can't lift weights, you know. So, I've developed and designed different ways to do things, probably not the most traditional way, but they work. And so I help people find ways to do things they couldn't do before. . . . I always tell people that, you know, it's not just about going to the gym, or staying in shape, hand-cycling, and working out. It's about having a reason to get up in the morning." There's no excuse not to, says Hamill. A person with a major disability has to find a way to keep active and get their heart rate up regularly, otherwise "you're not going to have the quality of life that you want to. You're probably gonna have health problems, and you're not gonna last as long."

As do many para and most tetraplegics, Hammill has continuing issues with regulating body heat. His injury interferes with the capability of the sympathetic nervous system—the one responsible for most autonomic bodily functions—to send messages. "The first time I [got feverish from temperature dysregulation] was years after my accident and I was wheeling out on a track in Port Huron, Michigan, hand-wheeling my chair, trying to get my endurance up, on an 85 degree day and humidity. And I didn't realize I was getting lightheaded, and I was getting hot. I was just trying to finish my laps. And all of a sudden I woke up an hour later out in the middle of the track. I literally had heat stroke and didn't realize it. Oh my gosh. Luckily, I didn't die. And that was my first time experiencing it. And I'm like, 'What is this?' So, I talked to my doctor. I knew about it, but I didn't realize how or why it affected you. And it literally will get your blood too warm and gives your body a fever. And you get tired, lackadaisical, lethargic, you just [feel] exhausted." After that, Hamill has had a few other close calls, particularly in the summertime when it's over 80 degrees Fahrenheit, but he now is careful to avoid these situations and, if he is in a hot environment, carries a spray bottle to keep cool.

At the end of our conversation, Hamill tells me the reason he wanted to talk with me was the horse connection. He recently moved back to Michigan with his wife and their twin girls, close to where his family still owns the 145-acre Crazy Horse Stables, where he grew up. His children have started riding and they keep pestering him to go with them. "I tell them that I would love to ride. But I would have to be strapped in, and as much as I trust the horse, something can happen."

"Not for you," I agree.

Mohamed Kazamel, a neurology professor at the University of Alabama at Birmingham's School of Medicine, a clinician, and informal director of its new autonomic testing laboratory, the seventh such a lab in the United States and the only comprehensive one in the Southeast, is busy. He schedules our conversation for his lunch hour, and after the first thirty minutes have gone by, asks me to hold on while he goes out to the waiting room to tell a patient he will be just a little longer. I've contacted him so he can show me his rare thermoregulatory sweat test (TST) equipment, which can map exactly where a person's sweat glands are working and where they aren't. And I want him to explain to me why something that seems so trivial—the ability to ooze a watery substance through our pores—is in fact so important that when someone can't sweat, as Hammill experienced on that hot day in Michigan, they must be constantly vigilant or risk dying.

The first thing Kazamel does is show me the TST booth, which he refers to, slightly ominously, as a sweat chamber. It is a small glassed-in box in the middle of the room, eleven feet long, four feet wide, and nine feet high, with a table in the middle. Patients strip down to their skivvies, lie down, and a technician dusts them from neck to toes with a yellow indicator powder—a mixture of alizarin red, corn starch, and sodium carbonate. Then the ordeal begins. The technician leaves and activates two long infrared heat lamps overhead, slowly increasing the temperature. A steamer in the back keeps the humidity at about 48 percent, "less humid than the weather outside here in Alabama," Kazamel laughs. "The goal of the humidity is to prevent skin burns, because if the infrared lamps start to heat the room without water in the air, [it] is going to be bad for the skin of the patients." Six sensors placed on the patient and on the heat lamps monitor the temperature; the goal is to raise the overall body reading by about one degree to 38.5 degrees Celsius or 101.3 degrees Fahrenheit. Everyone is different, but usually within a half hour most people break into a full-body sweat, turning the powder from yellow to a deep purple or violet. Cameras on the ceiling snap photographs every five minutes. "We start getting these pictures, analyzing them, and looking up which areas of the patient's body do not sweat," Kazamel says. "We see mainly two types of patients: those who have problems in the brain and the central nervous system and those who have problems in the peripheral nerves, mainly the small nerve fibers that are supplying the sweat glands."

Depending on the patient's ailment, different color patterns will appear. Diabetics, who are often affected by neuropathy, pain or numbness in the nerves of the extremities, which recent research links to inflammation from reactive oxygen species, often show a "stocking and glove" effect. Spinal cord injuries may have no sweating below the injury site and excess sweating above. "When we get them inside the autonomic chamber," Kazamel says, "you will find a line of demarcation between the areas where they are able to sweat and not able to sweat. Interestingly, people who are not able to sweat over the lower part of their body because of a spinal cord injury—they are oversweating over their upper part of the body, and this is what really annoys them." Many of the other illnesses the lab sees are brain-related, since it is the hypothalamus that controls temperature. This includes brain tumors, multiple system atrophy (MSA), Parkinson's, and Lewy body dementia, as well as a genetic condition called anhidrosis, a complete absence of sweating.

The University of Alabama lab, which was designed and built in collaboration with Case Western University in Ohio, was quite inexpensive, costing only about $100,000, but took two and a half years to complete, opening in May 2018. It now sees five to six patients a day hailing from all over the South—Georgia, Mississippi, the Florida Panhandle, and even Arkansas. I asked Kazamel why there aren't more such centers. "Because you cannot buy them. . . . There are like two or three people who can build them in the country, engineering-wise. And then it is quite complicated. . . . There is a lot [to work through] with occupational safety, how do you get rid of the powder in the drain system, and all of that. So, although the idea is simple, it is not. But the main reason is that they are not available commercially. Nobody sells them. They have to be built on site."

To completely diagnose a sweating disorder, Kazamel tells me, the TST is often not enough. Usually it is complemented by another diagnostic tool, the quantitative sudomotor axon reflex test (QSART). "The thermoregulatory sweat test is the big sweat test. It applies the entire sweat output pathway from the hypothalamus in the brain, down to the brain stem, down to the spinal cord, and then to the nerves, and then to the small nerves, and then the sweat glands. So that's more of a comprehensive pathway assessment to the sweat, while the QSART assesses only the small nerve fibers and the sweat glands attached to them." In QSART, technicians place four electrodes or capsules on the patient's skin. These are filled with acetylcholine, a neurotransmitter, and administered a very mild electrical current for five minutes, which stimulates the sweat glands externally. If patients have abnormalities on both tests, this is generally because the sweat glands and/or the small nerve fibers attached to them are not working. In addition to diabetes, this can be caused by connective tissue disorders like Sjögren's and lupus. "But if they only have an abnormality on the TST, then the problem is likely to be in the brain. . . . While when we put them in the QSART, the four capsules are still able to produce sweat, because that's a local circuit. . . . A pattern of loss of sweat on the thermoregulatory test, and preserved sweat on the QSART is, I'm sorry, quite concerning for a central CNS diagnosis like multiple system atrophy, and a shortened survival."

These patients, Kazamel tells me, often have other autonomic nervous system issues, such as regulation of heart rate and blood pressure, phenomena that are all related to sweating. Exactly what I'd wanted to ask him about, after learning that endurance horses who do not have their electrolytes replaced can have heart arrhythmias and that those with spinal cord injuries can, as did Hamill, pass out in the heat. He explains: "If you cannot sweat in the heat, what's going to happen is that the other cooling mechanisms, including flushing of your skin [will be activated]. And when your blood goes to the skin, it escapes from the core of the body, depriving your heart of the amount of blood that it needs for the brain. You will also have static hypotension [low blood pressure] manifestations, which are dizziness, lightheadedness, brain fog. All of these are going to get even worse in the heat. Because the body is trying to cool down by sending most of its blood to the skin because it cannot sweat. So basically, the two functions of regulating blood pressure and heat regulation are quite interactive." Although it is rare with healthy people, this is the same process (and symptoms) that occurs during heat exhaustion: dizziness, muscle cramps, headache, nausea. If you experience any of those during exercise, stop! If untreated, they can lead to heatstroke, as befell a friend in his twenties while trail running in the Los Angeles hills after a night out. (Rest in peace, Liam.)

After this somber note, it's time to hear the good news about working up a sweat. But first, we need to understand something about how mito-chondria work, a topic that is so complex that I find myself with brain strain every time I talk to scientists who specialize in it. Mitochondria are organelles, little organs, inside cells enclosed in their own membrane and with their own DNA. (Fun fact: mitochondrial DNA is inherited only from the mother; the father's self-destructs after fertilizing the egg.) Mitochondria specialize in producing very high amounts of a molecule called adenosine triphosphate (ATP) from its counterpart, adenosine diphosphate (ADP). In fact, mitochondria help to convert ADP to ATP by an amount that is 10 billion times greater than what it would be if the cell were not alive. This difference represents a huge amount of potential energy, which is then used to accomplish other tasks in the cell. This is why ATP is known as the energy currency of cells. ATP does nothing except ferry that energy to where the cell needs it and then returns, as ADP, to be converted back to ATP and do it once again. The things cells need energy for are powering some chemical reactions, moving substances across membranes, and doing work. Cells that have higher energy demands—heart tissue, muscles, liver, brain, and sperm—have more mitochondria.

Mitochondria have both an outer membrane and an inner membrane. The outer membrane is porous, but the inner one is tightly sealed. Substances can only get across it with special transport proteins. This means that the contents of the space between the two membranes is very different from that of the space within the inner membrane, called the matrix. The space between the membranes has all sorts of small molecules, as well as partially processed glucose and fatty acids. Once inside the mitochondria, these latter two are both broken down by enzymes to an intermediate molecule, acetyl-CoA, which is the raw material for mitochondrial energy operations, accomplished by two interlocking chains of reactions, the tricarboxylic acid cycle, (TCA cycle; also called the Krebs cycle and citric acid cycle) and the electron transport chain. In the TCA cycle, a series of chemical reactions strips away the acetyl-CoA's electrons, giving them to two electron carrier molecules, NADH and FADH2, plus making a small amount of ATP. The NADH and FADH2 then transfer their electrons to the electron transport chain, which moves the electrons through a series of reactions ending with oxygen. The flow of these electrons is coupled to the pumping of positively charged hydrogen ions (protons) from the matrix by specialized proteins in the chain. This creates a gradient across the inner mitochondrial membrane—the protons want to get back across it, but can't. In a process analogous to a hydroelectric dam using the flow of water to generate electricity, another protein located in the membrane, ATP synthase, opens a channel to allow protons to flow back into the matrix, using that potential to drive the conversion of ADP to ATP. Because ATP creation is thus linked to the use of the proton gradient, which can range from a tiny trickle to all-out torrent, scientists describe it as coupled.

So what happens when demand for energy is high, say for instance on a rainy day when I decide to do burpees? I jump my legs into a plank, lunge them into a squat, and leap straight up into the air. Within seconds, I begin to pant and perspire. I breathe heavily because my body has already used up the small amount of ATP that was lying around in my muscle cells and now wants more—a lot more: ATP use can increase fifty to one-hundred-fold with aerobic exercise. This makes my mitochondria enter a vastly speeded up state, requiring much more fuel and oxygen and increasing the rates of all the processes described above to match the ATP rate needed to power my muscles. When I finally finish and collapse on the floor, all my systems are still revved up. Fuel supply to the mitochondria starts to gradually decrease, but is still high, yet ATP use is back to resting rates. When fuel supply exceeds ATP use, the mitochondria become "flooded" with electrons, which causes electrons to leak from the electron transport chain prematurely to form reactive oxygen species ROS), the molecules that can cause the inflammation that leads to disease.

Introducing the circuit breakers. After an exercise session, when the mitochondria have been in this very active state, the inner membrane activates one or more members of a family of proteins, the uncoupling proteins, and another, the adenine nucleotide translocases (ANTs), that are also embedded in the inner mitochondrial membrane. When activated, they unlink the proton gradient from the rate of energy production, making the inner mitochondrial membrane more porous, so protons outside of the inner membrane can re-enter even though they are not being used to create ATP. In the process, the energy normally used to produce ATP is released instead as heat, which is likely why intense workouts leave you with a glow and higher overall rate of calorie burn. The uncoupling proteins and ANTs also counter the production of ROS. So if you get hot and sweaty while exercising, embrace the bake. Your cells are getting a cleanse. Although scientists still have a lot to learn about it, one uncoupling protein, number three, appears to have an important role in skeletal muscles—it is only present in them, is stimulated by exertion, and has a very short half-life, just thirty minutes after you finish your last burpee, cursing and wondering why, if you run every day, it's so hard to do ten little jumps in the very same spot?

∞

Do you ever feel like the universe is trying to send you a message? And when you don't listen the first time, it politely taps you on the arm, clears its throat, and tries again? Such was the case on my whirlwind 2019 trip to Toronto to give a talk at the city's first ever Biennial of Art.

I was there to share my expertise on how the US military's research on combat rations has been used to create many of the consumer foods that line supermarket shelves and refrigerator cases. But the universe—and the public: only a few dozen people showed up—was largely indifferent to my topic. It had other things on its mind, like teaching me that no matter how deeply you may dive into history, there is always more to tell, most often the parts that we'd rather forget.

The day I arrived, Myung-Sun Kim, the Curator of Public Programming and Learning for the biennial, invited me to brunch at the Gladstone Hotel café in Toronto's Queen Street West neighborhood. After I'd nibbled my way through a heap of bespoke bacon, two orange-yolked local eggs, and mounds of savory, pan-fried potato cubes, she turned to me. "Tomorrow, I will begin with a land acknowledgment." I looked blank. She explained that in 2008, the prime minister apologized to Canada's Indigenous peoples for colonization of their land and the Indian Residential Schools. Since then, many organizations had started to do land acknowledgment statements, although there are many conflicting ideas about them. Less practiced in the US, she suggested I might be interested in reading more on my own if curious. I nodded and smiled, but I was too busy thinking about whether we should have people pick up a plate with samples of a canned stew and the entrée from a Meal, Ready to Eat (MRE), the US military's main field combat ration, as they took seats or pass platters later. When it came time for Kim's land acknowledgment at the beginning of the event, I was too busy remembering the cute little story I'd created about how difficult it was to get MREs to Canada to pay attention. And then, after the talk, a walk admiring the adorable bay-and-gable houses of Ossington Village and Little Portugal, a meal at La Cubana with my Cuban husband, and a bottle of wine, I promptly forgot about it.

Until the universe sent a second messenger. After arriving in Boston after a long day traveling during Toronto's biggest early November snowstorm ever, Rafi and I scrambled aboard the Silver Line bus, which circles the airport, crosses Boston Harbor in the Ted Williams Tunnel, and deposits passengers in South Station, the downtown train and bus hub. I teetered in the aisle for a few moments until a low, sweet voice behind me said, "Sit." A white-haired woman, in a dark quilted jacket, slacks, and an immaculate handbag gestured to the seat beside her. I plopped down. "Feels good, doesn't it?" she said. I felt a quick pang of grief. My mother, who'd died two years earlier, might have said something similar.

"Where are you coming from?" she continued.

"Toronto. How about you?"

"Oh, I'm just riding the bus," she said. "There for some kind of event?"

I told her about the biennial and about the talk I'd given about my book. "There are so many influences," I said. "Tinfoil, for example, was invented by the Reynolds Company from tin ingot made from surplus jet planes after World War II. Or M&Ms. A member of the Mars family went to Europe scouting for candy treats to offer to the military and found something like them in Spain—chocolate inside a hard sugar coating." She made appropriate sounds of interest. "And I bet you didn't know that the Defense Department laboratory that does the research on rations is right here in Natick," a city a fifteen-minute drive away.

"Natick?" Her lips curved gently. "Natick means 'our home' in Algonquin. It was a village for the Prayer Indians, organized by John Eliot. Then, in 1675, the colonists wanted their land and shipped them off to Deer Island, where most of them died the very first winter." Okay, universe, duly chastened.

When we arrived at South Station, I extended my hand. "Thank you for a lovely conversation." Then I followed the stream of other passengers toward the train, for which, since we'd come from the bus tunnel under the Seaport, we didn't have to pay an entrance fee. I looked back and saw her straighten her thin shoulders in her winter coat, then set out for her destination. I realized that she had figured out that walking from Chelsea to catch the free airport shuttle was a way to avoid paying a $2.70 subway fare, and that she must be very hard up indeed. I wished I'd asked her name, and momentarily imagined her bright spirit alighting nightly on the bus, enjoying a lively conversation with another traveler. And then I went home to do the job the universe wanted me to do: to research the Indigenous history of Natick and the US Army Natick Soldier Research, Development, and Engineering Center site and create an unauthorized land acknowledgment on its behalf.

A similar erasure has happened with running. Before incursions by Vikings, English settlers, French traders, and Spanish explorers, the Americas—North, Central, South, and let's throw in the Caribbean for good measure—were held together by footpaths traversed by Indigenous runners. "These little trails, they're like webs that connect each of the villages together," Gilbert says. "And Hopi believe that they are like veins, their veins, and when the Hopi runs on these trails, they are bringing this much needed life through the veins to keep the villages alive." The southwestern United States is home to some spectacular distance athletes, but running was part and parcel of the fabric of tribal life everywhere, from the Rhode Island Narrangansetts and Novia Scotia Micmacs to the Sac and Fox Nation of Oklahoma, Pueblos of New Mexico, and Yurok of Northern California. It allowed food to be gathered, hunted, or grown at remote distances—Gilbert talks about farmers running to fields forty miles away, laboring all day, then returning home at night; it was a communications network; it was a form of mental and physical training, encouraged among children and celebrated with ceremonial races; and, most importantly, it was a form of prayer, connecting runners to their pasts, to their communities, to nature, and to higher powers.

"What we're seeing now is a desire to return to the ancient ways of our people," Gilbert says. "And if we could do that, even just a little bit, we would be so much more grounded in who we are as Native people. We would see a connection to all of humanity that we may not have experienced or seen before. And we would certainly see a connection—less of a focus on ourselves and more of a focus on the greater whole, the community that each of us belong to. . . . [But] running is not just a Native thing. We are all runners, regardless of our history and our culture, whether our peoples originated here in North America, or in Africa or Australia, or wherever. Every one of us comes from a people of distance runners. And it's really up to us and our responsibility to learn about that and to find that past and make use of it in our lives."

9

Bats, Babies, and Immunity

There are few things as frightening as being jolted awake by screaming. If you are a parent, and it is your child doing the screaming, even worse. Several springs ago, just as the New England weather softened into a moist hug, the heart-stopping shriek of Gabriela, then in her early teens, pierced the night. Rafi and I ran upstairs to the attic. Gabi stood outside the closed door to her bedroom.

"A bat! There's a bat in my room," she blubbered. Across the landing, Mariela's pillow-creased face popped out groggily. Rafi and I opened the door a crack and slipped in. The overhead light was on, and a little brown bat circled the room frantically, its erratic flight suggesting desperation. Gabi had opened her windows, which, since it was still May, did not yet have their screens.

"Let's just leave. It will fly out eventually," I said. "Do you want to sleep in Esme's room?" The bedroom, right next to ours, had been unoccupied since she went to college.

"No," Gabi cried. "Get it out. I don't want it in my room."

As I patted her on the back, Rafi charged downstairs. "It's okay, sweetie. It won't hurt you. Bats don't usually bite people, and they don't get tangled in your hair. That's a myth. It's probably more scared of you than you are of it."

She continued to wail. It was a school night, and I began to scroll through all the things we needed to do the next day—classes, extracurricular activities, writing and consulting deadlines. We needed to calm her down and get everyone back to bed. Rafi reappeared with the broom, and I stepped aside so he could ease back into the room. He would use the bristles to nudge the bat toward the window. Then I heard a thwack. And another.

Mariela burst into tears. "No! No!" But it was too late.

"Get me a garbage bag," Rafi ordered. I obeyed, also grabbing two single-use grocery bags, a roll of paper towel, and disinfectant. I handed him the garbage bag, which he used as a mitt to grab and envelop the small, crushed body. I sprayed and scrubbed the spot where the bat had lain, then put the used paper towels into one of the grocery bags, knotted it, placed it in the second one, knotted it, and handed it to Rafi. I didn't say anything. I hadn't expected him to kill it, but I hadn't asked either.

Mariela was still on the landing when we came out, her eyes swollen from crying. I embraced her silently, hiding my tears behind her back. The little bat had one life, and we had taken it.

Like most people, I am inexcusably ignorant about bats. That changed with the coronavirus pandemic. As politicians, public health officials, and the press sought a scapegoat, one story riveted us: the Huanan Seafood Wholesale Market, a so-called wet market in Wuhan, China, where customers could procure seventy-five species of live, wild animals such as snakes, civets, and baby crocodiles for a special feast or supposedly curative dish. (This section of the market was closed in May 2020.) Horseshoe bats, widespread in Asia, aren't usually on the menu, but they can infect intermediate hosts in the wild. When these are caught and held in small cages for sale and on-site slaughter, they create the perfect conditions for the spread of disease. But what intrigued me about the story wasn't reconstructing the path the microbes took in their journey to human hosts, but that fact that something that could cause such severe symptoms in people—fever, cough, and difficulty breathing, proceeding to, in some cases, respiratory failure and death—didn't bother bats one bit. What was it about bats that made them so resistant to disease? I began to learn all I could about them.

Animals that don't move as we expect—parachuting spiders, slithering snakes, and, yes, what at first glance appear to be mice or rats on wings—terrify us. When I was six years old, this was the cause of a gratuitous bike crash. Feeling a tickling on my thigh, I glanced down and saw an itsy bitsy, white spider. I screamed, threw up my arms, and ended up in a twisted heap with my Huffy. My fright was a blow to my father who, believing fears should be faced head on, had his three young children jump off cliffs and rope swings into quarries and rivers, swim through pitch-black underwater tunnels, and catch snakes with our bare hands—"behind the jaw so they can't bite you." (Once, during a long car trip, when he'd stopped for an en plein air bathroom break, I saw a snake by the side of the road and proudly brought it to him. "Put that down!" he yelped as he zipped up his pants. "Rattlesnake!") Following his example, I've tried to rid myself of these visceral aversions and to help my children do so, too, but so far, the only tangible result is that I am the designated insect remover, a service I perform with a Tupperware bowl and a sheet of paper. Besides, I have to admit, our instinctual antipathy makes good evolutionary sense: these creatures could sneak up on us.

Bats unnerve us for other reasons than their odd locomotion. They are nocturnal, emerging under cover of darkness to feed, usually on fruit or insects, but occasionally on animals, including us. Although only three of 1,300 species (bats represent 20 percent of all mammal species) are parasites, vampire bats, named for a Black Plague–era legend, loom large in the human imagination. The bloodsuckers, which are only found in Central and South America, are actually miniscule—their bodies are from one to three inches long, and while they will occasionally attach themselves to a slumbering *Homo sapiens*, their more usual fare is cows and horses, which, lacking flexible arms and hands to wave about, cannot easily detach them. Left undisturbed, they feed for about twenty minutes, imbibing a mere tablespoon of blood.

Another unsettling chiropter trait is sleeping upside down. For this activity, bats prefer cave ceilings, the undersides of bridges, abandoned or infrequently used buildings, and, of course, tree limbs. The logo for Bacardí rum, a staple in the Salcedo household and at our mojito-fueled gatherings, was inspired by the sugarcane-pollinating fruit bats that occupied the rafters of the company's original distillery in Santiago de Cuba. Stylized versions aside, most people would hardly call bats cute. They have rodent-like bodies capped by compact, dark faces; enormous ears; and sharp teeth. Their immense, collapsible wings resemble brown or black umbrellas; adapted finger bones are the spokes to which is pegged a leathery membrane. And, finally, it is true that bats carry many diseases, from rabies to Ebola, Marburg, SARS, and most recently, the virus that causes COVID-19.

But as I found out more about them, the less eerie and the more interesting bats seemed. Fun facts abounded, such as hanging bats swivel upright to pee and poop so as not to mess themselves. And I couldn't help but notice that most people who worked with them described them with adjectives such as *amazing, incredible, intelligent, social,* and, most frequently, *misunderstood*. So I contacted a place that could explain their appeal, Bat World Sanctuary in Weatherford, Texas.

Weatherford is not the place you'd expect to find the world's largest bat rescue center. The late nineteenth-century town, about twenty-five miles west of Fort Worth, oozes charm. In July, upward of sixty thousand visitors descend on the Parker County Peach Festival; the rest of the year, they admire gracious Queen Anne and Victorian homes, enjoy antique stores and cafés, and stroll in Chandor Gardens, a subtropical paradise combining Chinese architecture with formal English flowerbeds. Bat World Sanctuary is located just down the street from the botanical garden, on a ramshackle property without a sign. The low, slope-roofed building—mostly paid for with $13,000 in crowdsourced funding—is putty-colored, with few windows. Inside swirls a separate bat-centered universe. In addition to offices, a kitchen, a clinic, and recovery and quarantine rooms, there are separate zones for fruit and insectivorous bats.

Addison McCool, Bat World Sanctuary's executive director, is a vivacious young woman who loves animals. One Sunday she gives me two Zoom tours—one during the day, when the bats are snoozing, and another at night, when they are active. We spend most of our time with the fruit bats, who are much larger, and, with their pointy muzzles, resemble flying puppies. The whole time we talk, McCool directs a constant, cooing patter at the bats, who squeak at her, flap their wings at her, and approach her from the ceiling or the air. "No, honey. No, honey. I know I taste like melon. You want cantaloupe?" she asks, removing a piece from the treat pouch at her waist. She shows me a 25 × 40 foot indoor enclosure and a 32 × 42 foot indoor-outdoor one; both allow continuous flying. The spaces are draped with hammocks, vines, ropes, and enrichment toys and puzzles; the padded floor has a special paint to facilitate daily cleaning. In the middle of the indoor enclosure is a large fake palm tree from which food—apples, bananas, grapes, and melon chunks—dangles. (The insectivores, not to be outdone, get regular mealworms and their own mock cave.) "Aren't you worried about disease?" I ask McCool, as she strokes a bat that's alit on her palm, thinking of my assiduous disinfection of the dark, wet spot on my daughter's bedroom floor. She shakes her head. "Since these guys [the fruit bats] were all born in captivity and have been in captivity their whole life, there's a lot less of a struggle with that. Now, the native species, obviously those are rabies vector species for the US. But, of course, everyone here is fully vaccinated, so we can handle them."

The sanctuary is a monument to the power of the human-animal bond. One day in October 1988, its founder, Amanda Lollar, left the Mineral Wells, Texas, furniture store she owned with her mother to deposit the day's earnings in the bank. On the sidewalk, she came across a Mexican free-tailed bat with a badly broken wing. Vermin. But she brought it back with her anyway and put it in a cardboard box with a slice of apple and some water—to die, she thought. To her surprise, it didn't. To care for her unexpected new pet, Lollar learned everything she could—there wasn't much—about rehabilitating bats, especially insectivorous ones. Sunshine, as the little free-tail was soon named, became Lollar's constant companion, inhabiting her pocket and living for one and half years more. "Even though this little, tiny being may be the size of an almond, it's as individual as people are," Lollar said in a 2018 interview with the Dodo, an animal stories website. Her love for Sunshine; the realization that bats, contrary to their spooky image, were clean, intelligent, and social; and the absence of knowledge and resources about their care set Lollar on a new life path—one she's adhered to for thirty-some years.

Lollar's first step was to convert the family store into the Bat World Sanctuary and Educational Center. She also promoted peaceful coexistence with the animals to Mineral Wells business owners by relocating bats in their buildings to over thirty freestanding boxes, built by her father, a retired army major. In 1993, when her mother passed away, Lollar sank her inheritance into a crumbling apartment building down the street, home to a large colony that the owner was threatening to exterminate. Once it was hers, Lollar turned its high-ceilinged rooms over to the resident thirty thousand Mexican free-tails. Her initial plan for the sanctuary had been to focus on injured native bats and return them to the wild, but "pretty soon after, people started coming to her and saying, 'We have these fruit bats that have nowhere to go. . . . They can't be released in the US, and they can't go back to their own countries,'" McCool says. (Fruit bats hail from the tropics.) The sanctuary now shelters over four hundred fruit bats and just one hundred insectivorous bats.

The dynamics of animal rescue—many of the fruit bats at Bat World Sanctuary are castoffs from zoos, the pet trade, and laboratories—attract passionate people. They are the heroes, and the facilities that don't, won't, or can't care for their bats properly are the villains. Lollar, McCool, staff, and other bat rescue organizations may be gentle with their tiny charges, but they are often fierce and strident about attacking those they believe have mistreated their animals. (These stories, replete with adorable bat videos, also make for gripping reading or viewing on social media, an important source of donations.) The recent acquisition of most of the bats from the Mini S. Exotic Zoo, a Mineola, Texas, roadside exhibit, is a case in point. In January 2020 the sanctuary got a call from Second Chances Wildlife Center in Louisville, Kentucky. Second Chances had agreed to purchase eight Egyptian fruit bats from the Mini S. Exotic Zoo, which had rave reviews from customers. "This place is awesome! Ever held a lemur? Ever had an otter sit on your lap? How about rub an anteater's belly? Well we did! And so much more. We had THE BEST time!" Sylvia H. enthused in an October 2019 TripAdvisor review. But when the Kentucky team arrived, they were horrified, according to McCool and Lollar's posts. The bat enclosure, which housed sixty animals, was tiny—a quarter of the size of a shipping container. The concrete building stank of ammonia, and there was no water. The only food was a yellow plastic dish of apple slices covered with bat droppings and crawling with roaches; it had been placed on the floor, making it difficult for bats, who eat hanging upside down from perches, to reach and consume. She says the Kentucky team didn't feel right leaving the rest of the colony, which the owner, Michelle Smith, a retired nurse, was planning to sell. Would Bat World Sanctuary take the remaining ten Egyptian fruit and forty-two Seba's short-tailed bats?

The Bat World Sanctuary crew jumped into action. Lollar immediately called Smith, who, in keeping with her description of the business as a "state-of-the-art exotic animal propagation, husbandry, and educational facility," expected compensation. Although its policy is not to encourage exotic pet breeders by paying for bats, the sanctuary, concerned about the welfare of the bats, shelled out the fee. Two days later, Lollar, McCool, and another staff member, Moriah Adams, drove two and a half hours east from Weatherford to Mineola. They say they were just as appalled by the squalid conditions of the bat pen as the Kentucky group—and further upset by the inappropriate carrying cases and sorry state of the animals in them. Smith had put the bats in wire crates, which do not provide comfortable perches—the wires can dig into the tender skin of the bats' inner claws. Some were injured. Several were pregnant, and others cuddled pups under their wings as they clung precariously to the fencing. They were all skinny and ravenous. As the Bat World Sanctuary staff loaded the cases into their van, they prodded Smith for detailed histories of their new wards. "And that's when we found out that one of the females, a sweet Egyptian, had recently given birth to a daughter, but that the zoo owners had sold her off as a pet." When they got back to Weatherford, the Bat World crew wrote a scathing online review of the Mini S. Zoo, accusing it of animal abuse.

They also made it their mission to track down the missing pup. "I just can't bear to imagine a bat all alone. They are such social, intelligent creatures," McCool says. After a week of badgering phone calls, emails, and texts, Smith yielded and gave them contact information for a man in Missouri. When Lollar called him, he was chagrined and agreed to surrender the baby, which he'd kept all alone in a birdcage. "Once he learned about the bonds these bats have with each other, he wanted to do the right thing and bring [her] back to her family," McCool says. After a quick once-over and spruce-up in the sanctuary clinic, they released her into the enclosure. "When we brought Lizzie back, she immediately gravitated towards one specific female. . . . They were cuddled up together, greeting each other, grooming each other. And she just stuck by this one female and she still does, so we're fairly certain that it's her mother. They're just the sweetest thing," McCool says.

"Bats tend to be really, really good mothers," explains Gary McCracken, professor of ecology and evolutionary biology at the University of Tennessee. "They live a very long time, and they have a very low reproductive rate, one baby a year, so they are very attentive to their offspring." Like many other warm-blooded animals, bats are born helpless. These two things are not unrelated: a constant, high internal temperature, called endothermy, is an evolutionary advantage. It maximizes the speed of enzymatic reactions and metabolic rate, allowing quick reproduction and growth, wide-ranging foraging, the ability to survive in a variety of climates and habitats, and, perhaps most importantly, a leg up in feeding and sheltering young. In bats, this starts before birth. Habits differ among types, but it is common to have a nursery, where pregnant and lactating females live to protect the young and support each other—even acting as each other's midwives. Infants, which are a quarter to a third of their mother's weight at birth, spend their early weeks on a couple square inches of warm fuzz, either suckling under their mothers' wings or tucked in her tail pouch. The bat mother's cozy body compensates for the newborn's greater heat loss and imperfect ability to regulate its temperature.

At night, when it's time for the mother to forage, there are two approaches. Some don't leave their young for a second: Baby latches onto mommy's nipple and hangs there like a clip-on ponytail while she visits fruit trees or gulps thousands of insects. Others depend on babysitters—a few moms who stay behind to mind a crèche, a mass of babies pressed together from the perimeter. Although each pair is reunited in the morning, occasionally "a bat baby will steal a bit of milk from someone else's mother," McCracken says. "Sometimes bat mothers will nurse other babies; they all take responsibility for ensuring that the pups are fed." Researchers have found that these roosting groups have permanent relationships. In McCracken's early work on Trinidad fruit bats, which roost in harems of fifteen to twenty females to one male, "what we found is that they were unrelated, but they stayed together their entire lives. They do stuff for each other." As I've talked with McCool and the other bat experts, I've detected a change in me. Bat faces—snub-nosed or long-snouted, over-shadowed by large eyes and ears—no longer look scary; they seem kind and intelligent. Their asymmetrical bodies—overdeveloped chest and arms—are no longer weird, just opposite to our own, with their long, dangling legs. And I'm incredibly touched and frankly awed by their devotion to each other, and especially to their babies.

Of course, like their human counterparts, not all female bats are cut out for motherhood—or trauma can interfere with their ability to parent. Such was the case with a tiny beat-up female, who arrived in late 2018 as part of what the Bat World Sanctuary calls "the Michigan 90," another rescue story that got them hot under the collar, resulting in online commentaries dripping with disgust for humans and their foibles. The Organization for Bat Conservation in Pontiac, Michigan, which had ridden to national and international recognition on the back of its tele-genic and charismatic leader, Rob Mies, was forced to abruptly close its doors. Mies was accused of sexually harassing a former employee, and, with the additional scrutiny of his activities, it was quickly discovered that he'd been overly free and easy with the finances. Bad enough. But far, far worse, at least in the eyes of Lollar and her staff, the bats did not seem to have been well cared for. Although it strained their resources, the sanctuary took in the fifty short-tailed fruit bats, ten Egyptian fruit bats, twelve African fruit bats, fifteen Jamaican fruit bats, two Indian flying foxes, and one Rodrigues fruit bat. As per their protocol, they neutered all of the males—except for one old-timer who was too frail to undergo anesthesia. The staff assumed the African fruit bat's weakened state meant he was no longer interested in carnal pleasures. Not so! However, his mate, who had been stressed by the events leading up to their arrival, wasn't ready for the consequences.

"We came in one morning, and found one of our resident female bats had a baby," recalls Adams in a Dodo YouTube video. "She started biting him. She definitely did not want Ronan." Although the pup, born in March 2019, was teeny—weighing just a few grams, sanctuary staff stepped in, at first feeding him single drops of milk through a silicone nipple, later several, and eventually tiny bits of fruit. They kept him warm and safe inside a "mommy roll," a towel sewn into a shape that resembles a mother's folded wing, invented by the Australian Meg Churches, a carer known as Battie Blue. But what the baby craved most was contact. "He really didn't want to be away from us at all," Adams says, and he would cry constantly when she was out of sight. After a few months, as he grew, they strung toys over his basket and he would reach for them, strengthening his muscles and honing his gross and fine-motor skills. Later, Adams would let him cling to her fingers as he excitedly flapped his wings in short sets, readying himself to fly.

When he finally took off, the Bat World Sanctuary staff transitioned him to the colony by placing him in the Geribatric Ward's treehouse—a sort of assisted living section for more elderly residents. There, Ronan could learn to be with his kind and train securely—the area has extra padding because some of the oldsters are unsteady on their wings. Once he was released into the main enclosure, Ronan quickly found his mother and, despite their early estrangement, "she accepted him back," McCool says. "They now hang out together every night—they're often side by side. They're very cute." The redemptive power of love, despite a troubled history.

∾

It takes a lifetime, at least for the less enlightened of us, to realize how much we are shaped by our childhoods. Which is why, in a book about my own battle with disease, I am a liar if I don't tell you how much of it is a reaction to my mother's struggle with hers. My mother, an only child, had fantasized about having a brood of ten, a number she whittled to four when she and my father began breeding in earnest. But after a relatively easy time with her first three—my brother, sister, and I were born within a four-year span: nothing. What's more, although she'd stopped nursing when Daphne was six months old, two years later, her periods still hadn't returned and her breasts dripped milk. Eventually, they talked to their obstetrician about it. Was this normal? No, it wasn't.

My parents' quest for a diagnosis took almost a decade. During that time, under the rambunctious life of our young family tapped the persistent rhythm of my mother visiting with this and that specialist, hushed and worried conversations with my father (when he was home, which was rarely), and a low-grade depression that clung to her like body odor. They didn't bother to shield me, their dark and solemn oldest daughter, from their concerns. I retreated into books and my own thoughts, which were increasingly filled with loss and death. What would happen if my mother died? When I was twelve or thirteen, an endocrinologist finally figured out what was wrong with her: she had a tumor in her pituitary, the master gland that controls all hormones. It could be treated with a very long course, possibly even a lifetime, of drugs, or it could be removed surgically. For my mother, it was an easy choice. She just wanted this intruder gone. But the first surgery failed. And so, a few years later, did the second. My mother still refused to take medication. Finally, her endocrinologist offered her an experimental treatment: Would she like to be one of the first patients on whom a proton beam was used to excise a tumor? Of course, there were risks, such as inadvertently damaging the gland, but . . . my mother didn't think twice.

The radiation therapy was a complete success, annihilating the tumor. Unfortunately, it also annihilated all of her pituitary function. So my mother's goal in having the treatment—to avoid taking medicine for years—was cruelly inverted: she would now have to take artificial hormones every single day of her life to replace the ones she could no longer produce naturally. This long episode was but the first chapter in my mother's book of illnesses and conditions, perhaps brought on by her hormonal imbalance and long-term steroid use. Always overweight, she became obese, developing heart disease. In her early fifties, she had a stroke. In her sixties, she was diagnosed with rheumatoid (and severe osteo) arthritis and, in her seventies, with Parkinson's. But other than a couple draconian diets, she mostly refused to take care of her body—to exercise it, groom it (the words *tweeze, trim, shave, brush, whiten*, and *moisturize* were not part of her vocabulary), or even to dress it nicely, as if she'd never forgiven it for its betrayal of her.

I was my mother's caregiver in her final years; it was the appropriate culmination of my lifetime of worry. Now, every time I went to bed, I wondered if she would make it through the night. I brought her to doctor's visits and to the emergency room. I filled her prescriptions and bought her medical supplies. I worked with a never-ending stream of nurses and home health aides. I joked, not very funnily, that she was my most demanding child, and I resented her impositions on my professional, creative, and family time. Her multiple illnesses were ever-present in my mind, as was her impending death, which I refused to acknowledge to myself, even as Rafi warned me, "Your mother is getting frailer and frailer. I don't think she has much time left." But most of all, I still lived in terror of losing her, my gentle North Star.

After she did die, I gradually became aware of something else mixed in with the intense grief: the fear I'd lived with all my life was gone. I'd been an anxious child, an insomniac. Now, I felt at peace and fell asleep without tossing and turning. My days had the normal frets and stresses: Would Mariela get her report—started on the due date—done on time? How did our bank account balance get so low when I just deposited a big check? Why did I waste time reading the news and shopping online when I should be doing what I always dreamed of doing, writing my book? Does my sister not like spending time with me; is that why she's always canceling trips we've planned for weeks at the last minute? I was shocked at how quickly my lifetime of worry receded. I was not the person I thought I was, neurotic and uptight. I was just a child whose mother had thoughtlessly left open the door as she cowered before her own decline and death, and I had been living in that room ever since.

Almost as soon as I was diagnosed with MS, I vowed not to react to it as my mother had to her brain tumor—by panicking, pausing my life, and searching futilely for a medical fix. When I became a parent, I doubled down on this approach. My mother had given free rein to her fear and low spirits, unintentionally infecting her children. I would hide my illness so my daughters would never spend nights fearing what would happen if their mother died. My mother put everything on hold as she waited for an answer. I would barrel ahead, refusing to take more minutes out of my life than absolutely necessary, even if that meant driving or running with a numb right foot and drinking ungodly amounts of coffee to stay my gratingly peppy self. My mother would spend years going to specialists to diagnose and remove her brain tumor, and then, when her later conditions and diseases developed, turn being a sick person into a full-time job. I would go it alone, eschewing the medical establishment except for the necessities, and look to a regimen of self-care to keep my functioning as good as it could be. Sometimes I ask my children, "Do you ever worry I'm going to die?" They look mystified. My greatest pride is the fact that they take me for granted.

∽

Our nighttime tour, done in infrared light so everything is black and white, is a lot rowdier than the daytime one. As soon as McCool cracks open the door to the fruit bat enclosure, she is greeted with loud calls from Coconut, a resident of the Geribatric Ward. His voice is deep and commanding, as befits a gentleman of his age—twenty-six, about one hundred or so in human years—and stature, the only unneutered male in the colony, a privilege he now refrains from exercising. McCool rushes over to give him a small piece of honeydew melon, which he rolls around in his somewhat toothless mouth until all that is left is a small, white pulp. Revived by this sustenance, Coconut climbs gingerly down from his perch—his days are spent dozing on a hammock with his elderly harem of six—and approaches the food tree, where he will while away another delightful evening, snacking and chatting with his two best friends, Egyptian fruit bats Ethel and Lucy. Although Coconut is one of the sanctuary's most senior members—the oldest is Statler, a thirty-three-year-old Indian flying bat, his lifespan is not unusual. Bats are known for their longevity, some four to eight times longer than other mammals their size. As McCool moves around, she is trailed by clouds of bats. In the background, some hang from the ceiling in little groups, others cluster at the fruit tree, but many others are just swooping back and forth. "Obviously, the elderly ones don't fly as much here. But the young ones do a lot of flight practice. I mean, they just go around and around," McCool says.

Birds are built for the air. Their light bones, dense feathers, and relatively large and powerful hearts allow them to take off quickly, glide and soar among the currents, hover or migrate thousands of miles, and stop on a dime. Mammals, on the other hand, are mostly earthbound—although a few patrol the ocean deep. To reverse engineer a breastfeeding fuzz ball for flight, nature had to scrap many standard operating features for our biological class and invent a host of snazzy, new ones. Backwards knees. Echolocation. Wings, that since they are essentially giant hands, can be flexed into an infinite number of shapes, making for extreme maneuverability. These last two gifts combine to create a frighteningly precise hit-to-kill guidance system. Insectivorous bats, some 70 percent of all bat species, are tiny missiles, leaving their roosts at dusk to lock onto, track, and munch out of thin air about eight thousand hapless mosquitos, beetles, moths, or other crunchy prey daily.

These all-night food fests make for a lot of miles, but surprisingly little research has been done on exactly how far they roam. Scientists at the Ecology and Biodiversity Department at the National Autonomous University of Mexico recently conducted a novel tracking study of the lesser long-nosed bats, some females of which migrate from California to the Sonoran Desert every summer to birth and nurse their young. These bats sip nectar from agave flowers (their pollination services keep the succulents healthy, for which tequila drinkers the world over are grateful) and other desert blooms—but to consume enough sugar water to meet their daily energy needs is a monumental quest.

To find out how far they flew to find food, the researchers dusted the noses of thousands of mother bats with different colored fluorescent powders as they emerged from their daytime roosts, then captured and released bats from known foraging sites, as well as examined excrement. Amazingly, these pregnant and lactating bats flew twenty-five to thirty-one miles from their nurseries, indicating round trips of at least fifty to more than sixty miles a night. "Beyond the 49 km traveled each way, this species hovers while feeding. This means that they are very likely capable of flying much longer distances while commuting or migrating," ends the write-up of this experiment. McCracken also did a project tracking the lesser long-nosed bats with a colleague, Tom Kunz, who died in 2020 of COVID-19. "If you look at the maps of bat flight we created, they basically confirm that bats are flying up to one hundred miles a night." Other tracking studies echo this, although not all species go so far from home. Following a small group of Panamanian long-legged bats revealed they travel twenty-two to twenty-nine miles a night to forage, and Trinidadian fruit bats, the first McCracken studied in his long career, only four to five miles. "They visit the same trees night after night. They pretty much know when a tree will be in bloom, and if there's a lot of food, they call all their friends." (Of course, these feats pale in comparison to birds. Migratory species such as the bar-tailed godwit, which summers in Alaska and winters in New Zealand, can fly for nine days over open ocean—more than six thousand miles—with no food or water. The Canadian avian biologist Christopher G. Guglielmo likens this to a human moonshot.)

I try to picture the equivalent amount of physical activity for a person. To fuel their nightly expeditions, for example, insectivorous bats of the northeastern United States need to eat a quarter of their body weight. That's the same as 24,375 calories for a 150-pound man. Although bats fly closer to their maximal rate of oxygenation, a trick allowed by running their metabolisms solely on fatty acids and proteins, we'll permit our guy—whose sprinting rapidly depletes the glucose it burns—to plod along at a fatty-acid and glucose-burning jog, four to six miles per hour. At a five-mile-per-hour pace, he will burn 119 calories a mile. So, if he's munched a quarter of his body weight, we'll allot 2,500 calories for his daytime activities (bats mostly doze) and 21,875 calories to spend on his nighttime travels. I enter everything into an online calculator and it spits out—ta-da—184 miles. So envision running four ultramarathons every night. Is their high level of physical activity the secret to bats' immunity to disease and remarkable longevity?

Some families bequeath good habits like regular attendance at houses of worship; sacrosanct Sunday dinners teeming with aunts, uncles, cousins, and grandparents; or a can-do attitude with chores, maintenance, and repairs. Not mine. Instead, we dabbled in alcoholism and were either explosive abusers or conflict-averse pushovers. But I did inherit something of lasting value: a three-generations-and-going-strong commitment to daily exercise.

It started with my paternal grandfather who had been a breaststroke champion and a lifeguard during the 1920s, when the Hudson River bobbed with several floating pools presided over by buff young men from the Washington Heights neighborhood in Manhattan. These experiences engendered in him a lifelong love of the sport. He swam at the 92nd Street

Y, but on the days he didn't, he walked—always dressed nattily in an overcoat, cashmere scarf, and good leather shoes. (Okay, in the latter years there were some sweat-suit ensembles, but my point is, the dude had style!) My father took up the baton with his daily runs, never less than five miles and often over ten. The legacy has been passed intact to me and my two siblings, who, although we all have different lifestyles (perfect suburban family, urban mess, and cool, retired bachelor), all exasperate our mates with our insistence on at least an hour of gym, yoga, running, or walking a day. I started running three months into my pregnancy with Gabriela when I injured my rotator cuff projectile vomiting. I'd used my right hand to prop myself up on the bathroom counter and twisted it violently when I began to gag into the toilet. Until then, my young-mom fitness routine was three to four early morning swims a week at a Boys and Girls Club in an adjacent city and inline-skating in the nearby schoolyard or along the river on the weekends. Now how would I get exercise?

Put on my sneakers, open the front door, and run. It was early spring, and a few forlorn snowdrops were poking out of the ground, still covered with patches of dirty snow. I ran north for a bit, then turned east, south, and west again, dodging slushy puddles and icy patches and heartened by a couple more clumps of snowdrops. I did not enjoy it. I felt heavy—a fact not helped by my three-month pregnancy—and was soon out of breath. But when I got home, I felt warm, energetic, and cheerful. The feeling stuck with me the entire day as I ferried Esme to her activities, emailed clients, did housework, and made dinner. Was this what they meant by runner's high? The next day, I went running again, going a little further. And the next, and the next, and the next. So began a habit that I've maintained now for twenty years.

After a while, I began to notice something—in addition to the fact that I felt frisky, nimble, and quick and, although I'd lost no weight, my pant size got smaller. When the inevitable colds, flu-like illnesses, and stomach bugs made the rounds in the winter, felling various family members, I seemed to be impervious. Of course, I still kept my distance from the afflicted, but while the girls, Rafi, and my mom were sniffling/sneezing/coughing/vomiting/spurting diarrhea, I would feel symptoms coming on—and then I'd go for my daily run, careful to go shorter and slower than usual so as not to overly stress my body. Afterward, I might have a mildly sore throat or feel peaky for a while and then—nothing. That was it. No illness—and no MS flare-up afterward. What the hell was going on?

∞

At nineteen, after losing a foolish game of apply-to-just-one-college roulette (Brown), I was unceremoniously dumped by the educational system into the real world. Fine, they didn't want me? I'd move in with my (older) boyfriend, who was completing his senior year in college, and his siblings, graduate students, all of whom shared an apartment. I got a job doing data entry, enrolled in a chemistry course, and volunteered for two jobs in what was then a possible career path, psychology. I became the youngest ever counselor for a hotline for parents who needed to calm down before they exploded or hurt their children, and I did research and wrote for a child abuse clinic at the Children's Hospital. I was happy. I felt like a real adult, inventing my own life, biking around to my various activities.

But after one long, rainy November commute, I felt truly awful and went to bed early. The next day, I couldn't get up. I had a high fever, chills, and couldn't eat. After a week, I wasn't better, but worse. Dave called my mother, who brought me home and to the doctor's, where I was diagnosed with Epstein-Barr virus (EBV) and hepatitis. No one could figure out how I'd gotten a blood-borne disease; I wasn't an intravenous drug user, my boyfriend was too busy studying astrophysics to be unfaithful, and I'd had no transfusions—the mostly likely source seemed to be the hospital blood laboratory, which shared facilities with the child abuse clinic.

I spent the next two months convalescing. My liver couldn't digest fats, so I subsisted on plain baked potatoes. I learned origami, and folded several zoos' worth of paper animals, some of which still grace my Christmas tree. And I applied to college again. In time, I recovered fully (although my relationship with my boyfriend didn't), enough to master chugging pints of draft beer with friends during a two-for-one happy hour special, a skill that came in handy the following year when I went to Columbia. I didn't give my strange illness another thought, except to humblebrag about how I'd had hepatitis—I thought it made me look louche, like a downtown musician or artist—and make jokes about how I hadn't thought it was possible for my already yellow skin to get any yellower.

But it turns out that I wasn't alone. Many multiple sclerosis patients report having had mononucleosis, which 90 percent of the time is caused by Epstein-Barr, a virus that, although it subsides, never departs, settling permanently in your nervous system. And if that weren't enough to suggest an association between MS and infection, while 90 percent of the general population has antibodies to EBV, 100 percent of MS patients do. A recent Harvard Chan School of Public Health study has confirmed this link and estimates that EBV infection increases your chance of getting the disease by a factor of thirty-two. The exact mechanism is still unknown; scientists speculate that they may already be genetically susceptible and that the viral illness primes their systems for the disease. Whatever. A few years later, when my MS began, I noticed that attacks always seemed to come after I'd had some kind of illness.

Doctors have suspected since at least the 1960s that there was a connection between viral infection and multiple sclerosis. From 1961 to 1963, Western Reserve School of Medical neurologists William A. Sibley and Joseph M. Foley did a study to see if vaccinations triggered disease exacerbations. They found no relationship. What they did find was that MS flare-ups came after runny noses, sore throats, coughs, and diarrhea, and, like the illnesses themselves, peaked in the early spring after months of being spread in classrooms and offices. Since then, the link between viral infections and disease course has only become clearer. Medical scientists now think that cytokines, signaling proteins that act like microscopic emergency flares and which are triggered by infections, migrate across the blood-brain barrier, attracting white blood cells to mistakenly destroy the myelin sheath, a casing for neurons that also acts as a transmitter.

I had added bats to this book for the same reason I enter all my subjects: curiosity. When I began my research, I knew shamefully little about them. I didn't know how ancient they were, that they were such a successful order—inhabiting almost all climates and with stunning diversity; that the funny-faced, little furballs dominated a form of movement that belongs to the birds; that they were incredibly social, living in large, harmonious groups that interact constantly and are loving and attentive parents. I knew nothing, except my habitual desire to look closely at what other people deem disgusting or disturbing and bats' alleged role in originating the devastating COVID-19 pandemic that, in the United States, fueled by the incompetence and indifference of American leadership, was essentially a geriatric genocide. I was deeply perturbed, and worried that, in a misguided attempt to eradicate the purported cause of the pandemic, people would push to exterminate bat colonies. (Of course, this would root out nothing. We would still be vulnerable to viruses caught by domestic pigs and poultry, wild animals, and the insect-borne illnesses, spreading with their expanded ranges, the product of climate change.) I hoped my exploration of why bats don't get sick from the illnesses they impart to humans and how they arrived at such old age might help shield them against a scapegoating world. But I didn't expect to also find an answer to my quest to understand my own three-decades-long resistance to a disease that, for most people, is a sentence to increasing disability and, sometimes, early death. But here it was.

∞

I try to be charitable when Rafi gets sick. But either it's true that men and women have different pain thresholds—being slowly split open to pass a bowling-ball-sized object through your vagina is great training—or he's a hypochondriac. He complains pitifully. His throat feels weird when he swallows. He is congested. He is tired and achy. Can I feel his forehead? He's burning up! Where's the thermometer? Should he call the doctor or just go straight to the emergency room? I ride the wave of frustration that washes over me with gritted teeth and tell him I don't think it's serious and he should just rest. Living with MS has taught me to ignore dull aches, twinges, and odd sensations. The alternative is emotional quicksand: Is that a symptom coming on? Am I having an attack? Will it leave me permanently disabled? But Rafi has never had a brush with his own mortality and is as startled as a teenager when his body doesn't run perfectly. So I ask him how he's feeling, collect the snowstorm of used tissues strewn over the bed and floor, and remind him to drink water.

But I don't worry much about catching his bugs. Anymore.

My first multiple sclerosis attack, the stroke-like loss of strength and sensation in my right side, came after a virulent case of conjunctivitis—a perennial hazard for contact-lens wearers, who are constantly touching their eyes. So did my second, again stroke-like, but this time on the left side of my body. The third, fourth, and fifth, roughly every few years over the next decade, each affecting my legs, feet, and clitoris, came after flu-like illnesses, the kind that lay you up for days and leave you shaky and several pounds skinnier. As a mother, caretaker, and a small business owner, I invariably got up before I was fully recovered. Within days, my thighs, calves, and soles of my feet would throb with intermittent pins and needles, called paresthesia, a frequent MS symptom. After one of these illnesses, I not only had an MS attack, I broke out with intensely itchy red bumps all over one side of my abdomen—shingles. The condition, which is a recurrence of the chicken pox virus that forever after lives in your nervous system, emerges when your immune system is weakened. It is common among the elderly, but not for women in their thirties, as I was then. Although it wasn't part of the official care plan for multiple sclerosis, I noticed the pattern of illness followed by an exacerbation, becoming extremely paranoid about getting sick.

When I was taking care of my medically fragile mother, this was easy. She was my excuse. When I got word that a participant in a planned outing, an invitee to a birthday party, or a sleepover host wasn't feeling well, I'd cancel. The girls would howl in protest, but I was firm. "We don't want to get Nana sick," I'd say. "She might end up in the hospital again." Years before the COVID-19 pandemic, I was a stickler for copious handwashing, sneezing in elbows, and in-house quarantines the minute someone got a cold, flu, or stomach bug. The invalid would be confined to quarters, and I would deliver meals, water, aspirin, tissues, and thermometers, plunging into the stale-aired sickroom holding my breath. We were remarkably successful at keeping my mother from many of the inevitable school and activity-related contagions. (Although, yes, there were a few trips to the emergency room: once, while sick, she fainted coming down the stairs—Rafi, who was below, miraculously caught her, and once, after several days of vomiting and diarrhea, she became stuporous, responding to questions in a spacey tone. Electrolytic imbalances, both times.) But after she died, I had no other immunocompromised person to hide behind. I would have to ask people to miss highly anticipated events because of me, an idea that made me very uncomfortable, both because I feared disappointing those I loved and admitting my own vulnerability to them. Luckily, by then the girls were in their teens and less prone to school-spread illnesses. But I was also growing more confident that I wouldn't get sick at all, or, if I did, would get through it without an MS exacerbation. I didn't know why, but I knew the running I had become committed to in the ensuing years had something to do with it.

Bats' bodies are beautifully adapted to their regular feats of endurance. They are all powerful chest and sweeping wings (their length is why bats must hang upside-down, dive to start flying, and urinate by swinging upright) with shrunken abdomens and legs. Inside, there are lungs that are almost three quarters bigger than for other mammals of their size; in flight, the amount of air inhaled can increase ten to twenty times. Their hearts, which are the biggest in relative size of all mammals—1–2 percent of their body weight; for our 150-pound guy, that would be almost three to six times the size of the normal human heart—can beat over a thousand times per minute and have an extraordinarily rich network of capillaries, allowing them to meet a high demand for energy. Unlike other mammals, bats' veins have muscles that squeeze the blood back to the heart, a much faster system than those controlled, as is ours, by gravity and a system of locks. Their blood has more hematocrit than other mammals, boosting its oxygen-carrying capacity.

Bats are equally astounding at the metabolic level. Most mammals burn glucose when they must do all-out exertion, since turning fatty acids into energy takes too long—but the body cannot supply enough for a prolonged demand, so they quickly stop or slow their pace. But bats, like birds, burn only fatty acids when they do strenuous activity. During flight, their metabolic rates increase fifteen to sixteen times over, one of the highest multipliers for a warm-blooded animal. (For comparison's sake, the metabolic rates of running rodents increase about seven times above resting rate—and then they need to sleep after about twenty minutes of it—and of flying birds, just twice.) This roaring fire generates a huge amount of heat, most of which is dissipated through the bats' skin. Yet there is a small and sustained increase in internal temperature and the intense physical activity has other effects—the creation of harmful types of oxygen and free radicals, insufficient oxygen, depleted fuel stores, altered pH balance, and changes in chemical composition—that damage cells.

Heat-shock proteins (HSPs) to the rescue. HSPs are ancient and exist in all organisms, from bacteria to primates, suggesting how essential they are. Scientists consider them housekeeping molecules. HSPs patrol the body for misshapen proteins and refold them, relocate them, or, when the damage is beyond repair, take them apart. They were accidentally discovered by the Italian scientist Ferruccio Ritossa, who was doing experiments on fruit flies. Someone changed the temperature on the incubator, and the geneticist observed new RNA synthesis. He hypothesized that it might be in response to the increased heat. (His description of that moment is pure poetry: "It does not matter if this interpretation was true or false; it was a working link between imagination and reality, like love."[26]) Although different types of animals have different HSP baselines (constitutive HSPs), the levels of individual members increases in response to different stressors (inducible HSPs). Bats, which spend up to twelve hours in intense physical activity, have some of the highest known HSP levels. "Bats present a constitutive [heat shock response] HSR that is by far (hundreds of times) more intense and rapid than that of humans, being associated with a high core temperature. . . . This suggests HSP expression in bats could be . . . an important model to study stress resilience and longevity in general."

To learn more about bats and heat-shock proteins, I spoke with Aaron Trent Irving, an Australian virologist who moved to Singapore to work at Zhejiang University–University of Edinburgh Institute. There he met some bat immunologists, and quickly began to focus on chiropters. "[Bats] can handle viruses and don't get sick. . . . And the more

---

26 Ferruccio Ritossa, "Discovery of the Heat Shock Response," *Cell Stress Chaperones* 1, no. 2 (1996): 97.

we studied bats, the more intrigued we got—they're amazing animals," Irving says. "They don't get cancer. They generally don't have any signs of aging. They're incredibly long-lived but they don't actually look old. If you catch a bat in the wild, you can't tell what age it is." (Brandt's bats, with a body size of just one and a half to two inches, can live over forty years.) "And their metabolism—there's something unique about it, because they can fly all day long and they have no side effects of this really high level of metabolism. So we started looking genetically at what is different about them."

How heat-shock proteins affect immunity and longevity in bats is complex. "There are many different components and they all kind of add up. HSPs are just one thing," Irving explains. "The high level of HSPs keep the body from accumulating damaged protein. The body has an unfolded protein response (UPR) . . . [which] will detect unfolded proteins and the immune system will shut down that pathway. But if you have high levels of HSPs, they are continuously refolding [the damaged proteins], and that means the UPR won't kick in." This allows bats to coexist with the viruses they harbor without showing any effects. In the long term, this and other factors combine to give bats astonishingly long lives. "What's most important is that [bats] seem to have what we call healthy aging. They don't look old. If you catch a bat in the wild, if it's a baby, you can tell it's a baby. If it's a juvenile, you can tell it's a juvenile. Once it reaches the adult stage, if you catch a bat in the wild, you have no way of telling if it's two years old or twenty years old. They look exactly the same. It's only at the very end of their life that a bat will start to get some gray hair," Irving marvels.

Human heat-shock protein baselines are much lower than that of bats, but they are elevated in people who do vigorous exercise. "Marathon runners also have high levels of heat shock proteins," Irving says. "But I have to caution: many of the bats . . . are flying ten to twelve hours a day. Some of them travel 150 km in one day. So it's not like a little bit of high metabolic exercise. It's all day, every day, constant working-your-butt-off exercise." But even if most humans fall short of that high bar, a single exercise session has been shown to increase HSPs, and repeated ones, even more so and for a longer duration. In 2008 the British exercise physiologists Martin Whitham and Matthew Fortes found that a single twenty-four-minute run over a flat surface at 60 percent VO_2 max (a brisk pace) increased by 250 percent levels of one type of HSP. The increased amount of these proteins not only quashes the transitory effects of heat and other physical activity–related stressors; they are then available to modulate a variety of disease processes and viral infections. Exercise-induced HSPs guard against metabolic syndrome, diabetes, and insulin resistance; improve cardiovascular disease and prevent heart attacks; reduce hypertension; and slow aging. When people get an infectious disease, HSPs kick into high gear—and fever stimulates the production of more of them. But if there aren't enough baseline and induced HSPs, the body's defense falters. One theory on why COVID-19 was so lethal for the elderly and those with metabolic and cardiovascular problems is that these patients have impaired heat-shock responses—they do not produce enough HSPs to overcome viral cell damage, leading to an out-of-control inflammatory response, the so-called cytokine storms. A recent study in Sweden found that unfit people were significantly more likely to be hospitalized with COVID-19, confirming a British study's finding that those who are not physically active were 32 percent more likely to be severely ill.

For a long time, exercise was thought to be detrimental to those with multiple sclerosis. More than 130 years ago, ophthalmologist Wilhelm Uhthoff observed that four of one hundred MS patients developed lazy eye after physical activity. This transient neurological symptom, still unexplained, but linked to a rise in core body temperature was soon joined by others such as weakness, paresthesia, and fatigue. (I myself have experienced Uhthoff's phenomenon a couple times, which is why I always say no thanks to saunas, hot tubs, and Bikram yoga.) As a result, MS sufferers were advised to avoid overheating in general, and physical exertion in particular. That conventional wisdom is now being overturned. Some scientists have found that exercise both prevents and treats neurodegenerative diseases in animals and humans. Multiple sclerosis is a bit trickier; HSPs are found on the surface of brain and spinal cord lesions caused by the disease. This is undoubtedly because they are an integral part of the body's immune response to injury, but also may be because they are somehow involved in the immune dysregulation that causes the lesions in the first place. Whatever their role in inflammation, there is overwhelming evidence that exercise-induced HSPs improve immune function in normal subjects and a strong likelihood that they both forestall and control MS flare-ups. In particular, one exercise-induced HSP, HSP72 (the number represents its molecular weight), has been found to be so protective against heat and other stresses that it has been suggested as a possible therapy, if a pharmacological agent could be found to stimulate its production.

There's another clue, an epidemiological mystery that no one has yet figured out. Multiple sclerosis varies with latitude, becoming more prevalent the further north and south you go from the equator. When I was first diagnosed, in Quito, Ecuador, the neurologist said he'd never had a case in his practice, but knew about MS because he'd done his residency in Mexico City. Growing up in Cuba—where only the winter months aren't inferno hot, Rafi had never heard of the illness. Possible explanations have ranged from exposure to sunlight to overly clean environments, but the answer may actually be staring us in the face: heat-shock proteins. While no one has yet compared their levels in human subjects living in temperate versus tropical zones, veterinarians have with cows and goats. In hot climates, large mammals—this category would include humans—have higher levels of HSPs. So they may be less likely to get the viruses that trigger MS and better able to quell inflammation in general. (And if you ever need a motivation to run in the dog days of summer, scientists have found that exercising in heat compounds the expression of HSPs.)

There will probably never be a cure for multiple sclerosis. During periods that I am overextended or getting sick, it quickly reclaims its territory, sending cascades of warning tingles across my thighs, shins, and ankles and enveloping me in fatigue. I live in fear of an injury that lays me up, freeing it to deepen its incursion into my body. But meanwhile, no matter what the weather, no matter my physical or emotional state, no matter the upsets and setbacks of the day, I open the door and start jogging. My heart thuds; my breath rasps. Step by step, day by day, I outrun the disease that lurks within me.

∞

The black splotch on Gabriela's floor haunts me. Although in life there are no do-overs, at least I can pair this ugly memory with one that ends well. One June, many years ago when Esmerelda was little, she, my mother, and I went to stay for several days at our house in Vermont. When we arrived, I threw open all the windows, which did not yet have their screens. We had dinner, read children's books, and then went upstairs. A small bat was circling the bedroom, frantically looking for a way out. As I always do when faced with household crises without Rafi, I solved it with a minimum of physical force. I got a broom and gently ushered the creature to the open window. We watched quietly—my mother standing in the doorway with her hands resting on Esme's small shoulders, and I, clutching the dusty broom—as the little brown bat flitted back into the soft night of the Connecticut River Valley. I see her still, darting through the dark woods and along riverbanks, tailing mosquitoes, moths, and lightning bugs. At dawn, her belly and mammary glands full, she returns to her maternity colony and nuzzles awake her pup, who burrows under her warm wing.

10

The Exercise Diet

I secretly love January. The holidays, with their exuberance, excess, and so much additional work, conclude. The weather is a cold slap, and nature, a skeleton—branches; a few brown leaves; hardy squirrels and unflagging sparrows; rough, frozen ground. I don't bother to make any New Year's resolutions. Not because I break them, but by that point, I'm so eager to return to a regular routine that they are unnecessary. But this year, both because of the pandemic and this book, I do. I will make a conscious effort to replace food-and-alcohol-centered meals and parties with outdoor activities. That means instead of meeting my friend Rebecca at a café, we'll carry our paper cups and go for a walk. Pizza with my sister's family becomes a trail-running event. And instead of the blowout gatherings we have with our Spanish-speaking friends, we go for bundled-up, three-hour group hikes, led by a couple who recently did El Camino de Santiago. This is not to say, when we can, we won't also host dinner parties and evening soirées in the backyard. (Although these are looking iffy. A new neighbor called the cops on us twice last summer; the police, standing sheepishly at our picnic table, told us they were having trouble hearing which house merited the noise citation.) But when I can, I will try to balance meal-based socializing with undertakings that keep people moving as they converse.

In fact, changing what we emphasize in our daily lives is the single biggest thing we can do to improve our health. If you, after reading this book, find yourself persuaded that to have a healthy metabolism, your diet is far less important than your activity level, I invite you to follow the exercise diet. Take some of the considerable time you dedicate to thinking about, researching, shopping for, cooking, eating, and cleaning up after food, and invest it instead in new and fun ways to move your body. Make sure you get at least one hearty meal a day of aerobic exercise, where your heart rate goes up and your breathing accelerates. Supplement it with a variety of other sessions of moderate-level exertion, strength building, and work on balance and flexibility. You can do this at the gym or on a mat, but it's more fun—and easier—to do integrative exercise where activity is part of everyday tasks. Have a dog? They appreciate at least four ten- to fifteen-minute romps a day and would happily take more. Meet a colleague or business contact for a stroll to hash out a project. Bonus: walking actually increases your creativity. Instead of cocktails, grab your significant other and follow some YouTube yoga or dance instructions or go for a bike ride together. Meet friends to hike or play pickup soccer, football, or basketball. Kids are activity-idea geysers. Go to the playground. Toss a ball. Play hide and seek. Chase and tickle them! Dust your tallest shelves, mop your floors, and tidy your yard, choosing rakes and shovels instead of leaf and snowblowers (better for the environment and neighborly relations, too). Take a martial arts or boxing class. Swim, hike, play racquet sports. And of course, run.

To try to understand what I thought was an intractable human problem, the so-called obesity epidemic, I widened my lens to include our closest relatives on the tree of life, wondering how they might help us better understand ourselves. But surveying our relationship with other animals revealed something horrifying. Our sedentarism has infected almost all creatures in our orbit: inactive pets, cramped laboratory animals, penned food livestock, and work animals with an upswing in lifestyle illnesses, such as fat horses that get laminitis, crippling them. Even when we rescue bats, the wild animals who are nature's endurance athletes, they must sacrifice their nightly marathons. The only ones who've escaped the drag of our inactivity force field are the ones that live closest to us, the parasites. The word *animal* comes from *animalis*, which means "having breath." We breathe to supply our bodies with oxygen so they can move. Our negative impact on the natural world, including ourselves, is tragic.

It's time to return to our birthright of regular and frequently vigorous movement. This means not only figuring out ways that pets, laboratory subjects, livestock, and other animals can move about as if they were in their native habitats, but to address the many obstacles faced by those who've been left out of fitness trends: low-income families who lack access to outdoor space or the time to partake in exercise, communities of color, those living with disabilities or limited mobility, and elders. One of the hurdles many of these groups face, sadly, is the threat of violence, especially against women and Black and brown men. "It doesn't always feel safe to be out and about," López Coleman told me. "I have been trailed by the police when I was out on a run. I'm a female runner, so there's a lot of harassment that can come with that, that I've had to deal with. You know, I've been trailed by just a random guy following me while I was out on a run." In the worst-case scenario, this aggression may end as did Ahmaud Arbery's innocent Sunday jog or the steady drip of news items about women runners who are sexually assaulted or murdered.

This book gives a tiny sample of the hundreds of known profound impacts of physical activity at the metabolic, cellular, and molecular levels. It activates different pathways for glucose to enter muscle cells. It creates tiny drops of lipids next to the mitochondria for quick fuel. It increases the robustness of mitochondrial networks. And it has an anti-inflammatory effect, minimizing reactive oxygen species through uncoupling proteins and boosting the production of the heat-shock proteins that repair, relocate, or discard damaged proteins. My focus aligns with a new scientific discipline, omics, which yokes high-throughput techniques for identifying proteins to the ability to collect and analyze heretofore unheard-of amounts of data. In 2017, for the first time ever, the National Institutes of Health began a mammoth, multiyear, multi-institutional omics project to inventory and characterize the huge array of molecules—collected from both animal and human subjects—that are produced during exercise. The project includes ten sites for clinical studies in humans, seven sites for preclinical animal research, nine sites for chemical analysis, and five sites for consortium coordination. The COVID-19 pandemic has slightly delayed the clinical trials, but the laboratory work on animals is just coming to completion, and already offering numerous intriguing insights into exercise's short- and long-term benefits—and the messenger molecules that induce those changes. Three people mentioned in this book, Frank Booth, Laurie Goodyear, and Darrell Neufer, are part of this endeavor, called the Molecular Transducers of Physical Activity in Humans. I spoke to a couple more, Wendy Kohrt, a professor in the Division of Geriatric Medicine at the University of Colorado and the chair of the project's executive and steering committees, and Karyn Esser, a physiology professor at the University of Florida and consortium member, just before finishing, to catch up on the latest.

They are both extremely excited about the results of the animal studies. "We can sample many more tissues from the animals," Kohrt says. "So we'll know about blood, muscle, and fat from humans, but we'll know about heart, liver, lungs, brain, bone—all sorts of things from animals. And that's going to be really important for a couple of reasons: both to have a better understanding of how our systems communicate with each other and because we may discover some signaling factors that the brain [uses to] talk to all of these other organs." Esser, who works with rodents, is more detailed. "We took three different parts of the brain—hippocampus, hypothalamus, and the cortex. Obviously, we took some skeletal muscle and the usual candidates, you know, heart, lung, liver, fat, white fat, brown fat. . . . But for me, one of the biggest stories with this is that every single organ system changes. And some of the bigger changes are seen in things like the adrenal and the colon, of all things." I'm so intrigued that I interrupt her to ask how. "There are a lot of epidemiological studies that have pointed to the fact that if you're physically active, your probability of colon cancer is lower. And, I want to be real careful here, but, yes, we see things related to cell cycle, we see things related to inflammation. So some of the big players, in terms of exercise response beyond the expected metabolic changes, is inflammatory responses across a lot of tissues. For me, as a scientist, the thing that really strikes me is every organ responds and in large numbers—we're not talking ten or fifteen genes, we're talking hundreds, in some cases, thousands."

Kohrt tells me that one of the most surprising results they're seeing in the preclinical animal work is a sex difference in the impact of physical activity. "It's already piqued the interest of people within our consortium. It's made the clinical scientists much more keenly aware of how important it's going to be for us to make sure that the group that we assemble, the cohort we assemble, is truly across the age range and equal representation of women and men. . . . [And it] highlights the importance of studying sex differences. If exercise doesn't generate similar responses between women and men, we can't expect any drug to do that. It just emphasizes the importance of any potential therapeutic strategy being evaluated for effectiveness in women and men distinctly."

I ask both scientists what their takeaways from the project are. Kohrt is altruistic. She hopes that the results create the "scientific foundation for how and why exercise has these very potent benefits . . . so that it becomes a well-accepted therapeutic strategy to treat diseases." Esser is more personal. "I have to say, it's increased my training. Just watching the data coming out with the animals, I'm just like, okay, at my age, I need to get back to this. When you see the scope of the changes, it's like, okay, this is no joke. This is not just my muscles. This is my whole system."

∾

For the past ten years, after my still-unexplained bilateral hearing loss, my health—except for a few running or activity-related injuries—has been perfect. As did many, during the pandemic, I postponed my annual checkup to allow medical practitioners to focus on COVID-19 patients and to avoid catching it myself. But by the summer of 2021, I felt comfortable enough to schedule my physical. Most of my discussion with my doctor centered on the painful mask-related rash that I'd mistakenly slathered with topical steroids, resulting in skin that was addicted to the medicine and would not heal. At the end of our session, my physician said, "Why don't you get a hearing test? It's been a while." So a few months later, I entered the little soundproof metal box used for audiology exams. The technician hooked me up and beeped and buzzed at me for a bit, then played a recording of a man cycling through a series of short words. I didn't get everything; I am, after all, deaf in the upper frequencies. Afterward, the technician slid open the door to the booth and began talking to me in an exaggeratedly loud voice. I had lost more of my hearing in the upper range on one side and in the middle range on the other. But even worse, my speech recognition scores had dropped to 48 percent in one ear and 40 percent in the other, a level that would qualify me as disabled by federal law. Suddenly I realized that what I had thought was a general quieting of the world outside my house due to the pandemic and the fact that the birds had all migrated south for the winter was a precipitous worsening of my deafness. "Maybe it's age-related?" I asked hopefully. "No," the audiologist stated flatly. Shaken, I immediately contacted my primary care provider, who arranged for me to see a neurotologist, someone who specializes in the neurology of hearing, at Massachusetts Eye and Ear Hospital.

Before our appointment, Dr. Felipe Santos read my MS case history, my hearing-loss case history, reviewed the results of blood and other tests, and ordered an MRI to see if there'd been any progression since my last one in 2011. (The attending radiologist for the MRI didn't even bother talking to me; he pantomimed for me to follow him to the radiology room and waved to a hook for me to hang my mask and locker key.) Santos got right to the point: this could still be MS, but it's acting an awful lot like another disease, Susac syndrome, which is actually an autoimmune system attack on the tiny blood vessels that line some organs, causing very small strokes. Although there were differences—Susac-related hearing loss is mostly in the low, not the high, frequencies, and it doesn't generally have spinal-column involvement, as I have had, this made intuitive sense to me. I'd long wondered if my atypical MS course, migraines with aura, and hearing loss was something else, maybe something with a vascular origin. Then he explained that Susac syndrome has a classic triad of symptoms: Swiss cheese–like holes in the corpus callosum area of the brain (check), bilateral sudden sensorineural hearing loss (check), and blindness (gulp). If it was Susac, and my hearing loss was progressing rapidly, he recommended treatment with prednisone and immune-suppressing drugs. If it wasn't, and possibly even now to preserve what I have left, I might want to consider cochlear implants.

I drove home stunned. I was already finding large gatherings difficult—I had trouble hearing the banter and often simply sat, entombed in my clanging tinnitus. At our impromptu Christmas Eve party, the din of the table drowned out Miriam's voice although she was seated right next to me; I watched her mouth nothingness. Now I imagined a future in which I can no longer see or hear the people I love. For the first time, I wondered if I could stand going through this. I felt my grip loosen on the steering wheel. When I got home, I shouted hello to Rafi and sat down in my office chair to research euthanasia, currently legal in two states. Could my cousin, who's a nurse practitioner, visit to administer me the fatal dose in Vermont, the perfect place to close the circle of my life? That night, in the darkness, when I sensed Rafi's wakefulness, I say quietly, "I might not want to be here anymore."

"What do you mean?" he says.

"Here," I say. "On earth."

Of course, in the morning, the moment of despair has passed. I know that no matter how difficult my existence is, I am bound here. It is the promise a parent implicitly makes in bringing children into the world: to always be there for them, loving, protecting, guiding, and bravely illuminating the path ahead. It's a promise I extracted from my mother when I sensed her crippled body dragging her toward the other side, and now it would be my turn. In her final years, she would wake up and say to me, wonder in her creaky voice, "I ran through a meadow in my dream." I pictured her, her limbs pain-free, strong, and flexible, barely touching the flower and grass-filled fields of her New England childhood. A few days later, I share my possible new diagnosis and my moment of midnight anguish with my friend Rebecca, whose birdlike voice is one of the hardest for me to understand. She doesn't offer sympathy. "What do you love?" she demands. "Whatever it is: do it." I don't say anything. But I see myself in a blur of motion, feet churning, heart throbbing, heat rising, the color wash of houses, the glory of the sky, the steadfast presence of the trees and animals, my thoughts flowing like water.

Footnotes

1. Ilya Kister et al., "Disability in Multiple Sclerosis: A Reference for Patients and Clinicians," *Neurology* 80, no. 11 (2013): 1018–24.
2. Vijayshree Yadav et al., "Low-Fat, Plant-Based Diet in Multiple Sclerosis: A Randomized Controlled Trial," *Multiple Sclerosis and Related Disorders* 9 (2016): 80–90.
3. Bianca Weinstock-Guttman et al., "Serum Lipid Profiles Are Associated with Disability and MRI Outcomes in Multiple Sclerosis," *Journal of Neuroinflammation* 8, art. 127 (2011): 127.
4. Marie Beatrice D'Hooghe, Guy Nagels, Véronique Bissay, and Jaques De Keyser, "Modifiable Factors Influencing Relapses and Disability in Multiple Sclerosis," *Multiple Sclerosis: Clinical and Laboratory Research* 16, no. 7 (2010): 773–85.
5. https://www.fda.gov/food/food-additives-petitions/food-additive-status-list
6. Laurie J. Goodyear, Michael F. Hirshman, and Edward S. Horton, "Exercise-Induced Translocation of Skeletal Muscle Glucose Transporters," *American Journal of Physiology* 261, no. 6 (1991): E798–99.
7. https://www.youtube.com/watch?v=5WHKZrGaSJo, around minute 8:30.
8. Among Lathrop's many unrecognized scientific and technological achievements is the invention of the cage water bottle. "On some of the cages, Miss Lathrop had rigged a device for giving them water. It is a bottle with a feed tube, from which a drop constantly hangs down into the cage, and a thirsty mouse has only to stand on his hind legs to quaff a cooling drink." *Springfield (MA) Sunday Republican*, October 5, 1913.
9. The patented JAX breeding method to prevent genetic drift in their mouse strains, already inbred through at least twenty generations of parent-offspring or brother-and-sister matings, is to refresh a naturally breeding colony from two "twin" founders every fifth generation with frozen embryos that are siblings of the original founders. This involves a short surgery to implant the embryos in a female who has been prepped for fertilization by having sex with a castrated male. Two offspring, a robust male and female, are chosen from this litter and placed in a box cage, where they will live a life of ease—no work, no danger, food and drink, and ample sex. Females will have their miniscule vaginas regularly examined with a toothpick or "blunt

metal probe" for "copulatory plugs," a cream-colored mass of mouse ejaculate. Her pregnancy can be confirmed eleven days after this has been discovered, and, if successful, will result in a litter of between two and twelve, who will also enjoy a carefree existence of making merry and whoopie. Repeat five times.

10. Agustin Zapata et al., "Microdialysis in Rodents," *Current Protocols in Neuroscience* (2009): unit 7.2.

11. US Department of Agriculture, "Tobacco Situation and Outlook Report Yearbook," Washington, DC, October 2007.

12. Ancel Keys, "Application for Research Grant," Council for Tobacco Research, New York, October 7, 1955.

13. E. S. Harlow, Memo to H. R. Hanmer, American Tobacco Company, July 19, 1956.

14. Ancel Keys and Francisco Grande, "Role of Dietary Fat in Human Nutrition, Diet and the Epidemiology of Coronary Heart Disease," *American Journal of Public Health* 47 (1957): 1520–30.

15. Martti Karvonen et al., "Cigarette Smoking, Serum-Cholesterol, Blood-Pressure, and Body Fatness Observations in Finland," *Lancet* 273, no. 7071 (1959): 494.

16. Ancel Keys et al., "Lesson from Serum Cholesterol Studies in Japan, Hawaii and Los Angeles," *Annals of Internal Medicine* 48, no. 1 (1958): 83–94.

17. Ancel Keys et al., *Epidemiological Studies Related to Coronary Heart Disease: Characteristics of Men Aged 40–59 in Seven Countries* (Tampere, Finland: Hämeen Kirjapaino Oy, 1966), 304.

18. Committee on Labor and Public Welfare, Subcommittee on Health, "Cigarette Smoking and Disease: Hearings before the Subcommittee on Health," 94th Cong., 2nd sess., May 27, 1976.

19. Ancel Keys et al., "Epidemiological Studies Related to Coronary Heart Disease: Characteristics of Men Aged 40–59 in Seven Countries," *Acta Medica Scandinavica* 460, suppl. (1967): 278.

20. Deposition of Henry Webster Blackburn Jr., MD, October 17, 1996, Mississippi Tobacco Litigation and Deposition of Henry Webster Blackburn Jr., MD, January 20, 1997, *Florida v. American Tobacco Company.*

21. *Botar la casa por la ventana* means "to throw the house through the window." It is used to describe the all-out attitude to entertainment common in Latin America and Spain.

22. Shari S. Bassuk and JoAnn E. Manson, "Epidemiological Evidence for the Role of Physical Activity in Reducing Risk of Type 2 Diabetes and Cardiovascular Disease," *Journal of Applied Physiology* 99, no. 3 (2005): 1193–1204.

23. I. Lehr Brisbin Jr. and Michael S. Sturek, "The Pigs of Ossabaw Island: A Case Study of the Application of Long-Term Data in Management Plan Development," In *Wild Pigs: Biology, Damage, Control Techniques and Management*-SRNL-RP-2009-00869, ed. John Mayer and I. Lehr Brisbin Jr. (Aiken, SC: Savannah River National Laboratory, 2009), 367.

24. Eugene Odom (1913–2002), a University of Georgia faculty member, is considered to be the father of modern ecology, with the publication of his 1953 book, *Fundamental of Ecology*.

25. Ossabaw Island's current incarnation, a gracious mansion in a wilderness preserve, cloaks an ugly past. The Indigenous Gaules were burned out of their village by the Spanish in 1579. After a period of relative quiet as a hunting and fishing preserve for English settlers, in 1763 John Morel, a colonist, brought thirty slaves there to farm and timber. Later, indigo and then cotton plantations were established; during the 1800s, these were owned by four families and worked by at least 160 slaves, who lived in cabins made of "tabby," a concrete made from crushed oyster shells and lime, three examples of which remain. After the Civil War, the island had a freedmen's settlement that established the Hinder Me Not African Baptist church. Many moved to the mainland community of Pinpoint after several devastating hurricanes in the late nineteenth century. The island was then purchased by the Torrey family, of which Eleanor West was a member, for $150,000. By the 1970s, the last remaining Black Ossabawans had abandoned the island.

26. Ferruccio Ritossa, "Discovery of the Heat Shock Response," *Cell Stress Chaperones* 1, no. 2 (1996): 97.

Sources

CHAPTER 1: POSTER CHILD FOR MULTIPLE SCLEROSIS

D'Hooghe, Marie Beatrice, Guy Nagels, Véronique Bissay, and Jaques De Keyser. "Modifiable Factors Influencing Relapses and Disability in Multiple Sclerosis." *Multiple Sclerosis: Clinical and Laboratory Research* 16, no. 7 (2010): 773–85.

Kister, Ilya, et al. "Disability in Multiple Sclerosis: A Reference for Patients and Clinicians." *Neurology* 80, no. 11 (2013): 1018–24.

Weinstock-Guttman, Bianca, et al. "Serum Lipid Profiles Are Associated with Disability and MRI Outcomes in Multiple Sclerosis." *Journal of Neuroinflammation* 8, art. 127 (2011).

Yadav, Vijayshree, et al. "Low-Fat, Plant-Based Diet in Multiple Sclerosis: A Randomized Controlled Trial." *Multiple Sclerosis and Related Disorders* 9 (2016): 80–90.

CHAPTER 2: FAT CATS AND DIABETIC DOGS

American Veterinary Medicine Association (AVMA). *2017–2018 AVMA Pet Ownership and Demographics Sourcebook.* Schaumburg, IL: AVMA, 2018.

Amiot, Catherine, Brock Bastian, and Pim Martens. "People and Companion Animals: It Takes Two to Tango." *BioScience* 66, no. 7 (2016): 552–60.

Axelsson, Erik, et al. "The Genomic Signature of Dog Domestication Reveals Adaptation to a Starch-Rich Diet." *Nature,* January 23, 2013, 360–64.

Baldwin, James Allen. "Notes and Speculations on the Domestication of the Cat in Egypt." *Anthropos* 70, no. 3-4 (1975): 428–48.

Canadian Veterinary Medical Association and Hill's Pet Nutrition. "Canada's Pet Wellness Report." Ottawa, Canada, 2011.

Clancy, Elizabeth A., and Andrew N. Rowan. "Companion Animal Demographics in the United States: A Historical Perspective." In *The State of the Animals II: 2003,* edited by Deborah J. Salem and Andrew N. Rowan, 9–26. Washington, DC: Humane Society Press, 2003.

Donoghue, Susan, and Janet M. Scarlett. "Diet and Feline Obesity." *Journal of Nutrition* 128, no. 12 (1998): 2776S–8S.

Diesel, Alleyn. "Felines and Female Divinities: The Association of Cats with Goddesses, Ancient and Contemporary." *Journal for the Study of Religion* 21, no. 1 (2008): 71–94.

Dye, Janice A., et al. "Elevated PBDE Levels in Pet Cats: Sentinels for Humans?" *Environmental Science & Technology* 41, no. 18 (2007): 6350–56.

Freeman, Lisa M., et al. "Diet-Associated Dilated Cardiomyopathy in Dogs: What Do We Know?" *Journal of the American Veterinary Medical Association* 253, no. 11 (2018): 1390–94.

Gagnon, Frank (psuedonym). Interview by the author. December 23, 2020.

Grimm, David. "Ancient Egyptians May Have Given Cats the Personality to Conquer the World." *Science*, June 19, 2017.

Guo,Weihong, et al. "High Polybrominated Diphenyl Ether Levels in California House Cats: House Dust a Primary Source?" *Environmental Toxicology and Chemistry* 31, no. 2 (2012): 301–6.

Horn, Jeff A., et al. "Home Range, Habitat Use, and Activity Patterns of Free-Roaming Domestic Cats." *Journal of Wildlife Management* 75, no. 5 (2011): 1177–85.

Hu, Yaowu, et al. "Earliest Evidence for Commensal Processes of Cat Domestication." *Proceedings of the National Academy of Sciences of the United States of America* 111, no. 1 (2014): 116–20.

Jenks, Susan. "Our Fat Pets." *New York Times*, August 2, 2018.

Karasov, William H., and Angela E. Douglas. "Comparative Digestive Physiology." *Comprehensive Physiology* 3, no. 2 (2013): 741–83.

Karlsson, Elinor. Interview by the author. January 12, 2021.

Kass Philip H., et al. "Evaluation of Environmental, Nutritional, and Host Factors in Cats with Hyperthyroidism." *Journal of Veterinary Internal Medicine* 13, no. 4 (1999): 323–29.

Kovaříková, Simona, Petr Maršálek, Monika Habánová, and Jarmila Konvalinová. "Serum Concentration of Bisphenol A in Elderly Cats and Its Association with Clinicopathological Findings." *Journal of Feline Medicine and Surgery* 23, no. 2 (2021): 105–14.

Ogechi, Imala, et al. "Pet Ownership and the Risk of Dying from Cardiovascular Disease Among Adults Without Major Chronic Medical Conditions." *High Blood Pressure & Cardiovascular Prevention* 23, no. 3 (2016): 245–53.

O'Neill, Dan G., et al. "Epidemiology of Diabetes Mellitus among 193,435 Cats Attending Primary-Care Veterinary Practices in England." *Journal of Veterinary Internal Medicine* 30, no. 4 (2016): 964–72.

Palmer, Clare, and Peter Sandøe. "For Their Own Good: Captive Cats and Routine Confinement." In *The Ethics of Captivity*, edited by Lori Gruen, 135–55. Oxford: Oxford University Press, 2014.

Pennisi, Elizabeth. "Diet Shaped Dog Domestication." *Science*, January 23, 2013.

Scarlett, Janet M., N. Sydney Moise, and Judith Rayl. "Feline Hyperthyroidism: A Descriptive and Case-Control Study." *Preventive Veterinary Medicine* 6, no. 4 (1988): 295–309.

Qureshi, Adnan I., Muhammad Zeeshan Memon, Gabriela Vazquez, and Muhammad Fareed K. Suri. "Cat Ownership and the Risk of Fatal Cardiovascular Diseases:

Results from the Second National Health and Nutrition Examination Study Mortality Follow-up Study." *Journal of Vascular and Interventional Neurology* 2, no. 1 (2009): 132–35.

Rowe, Elizabeth, et al. "Risk Factors Identified for Owner-Reported Feline Obesity at Around One Year of Age: Dry Diet and Indoor Lifestyle." *Preventive Veterinary Medicine* 121, no. 3-4 (2015): 273–81.

Thomas, Rebecca L., Philip J. Baker, and Mark D. E. Fellowes. "Ranging characteristics of the Domestic Cat (*Felis catus*) in an Urban Environment." *Urban Ecosystems* 17 (2014): 911–21.

US Food and Drug Administration. "FDA Investigation into Potential Link between Certain Diets and Canine Dilated Cardiomyopathy." Outbreaks and Advisories, June 27, 2019. FDA website. https://www.fda.gov/animal-veterinary/outbreaks -and-advisories/fda-investigation-potential-link-between-certain-diets-and -canine-dilated-cardiomyopathy.

Tan, Sarah M. L., Anastasia C. Stellato, and Lee Niel. "Uncontrolled Outdoor Access for Cats: An Assessment of Risks and Benefits." *Animals* 10, no. 2 (2020): 258.

Verbrugghe Adronie, and Myriam Hesta. "Cats and Carbohydrates: The Carnivore Fantasy?" *Veterinary Sciences* 4, no. 4 (2017): 55.

Weissengruber Gerald E., et al. "Hyoid Apparatus and Pharynx in the Lion (*Panthera leo*), Jaguar (*Panthera onca*), Tiger (*Panthera tigris*), Cheetah (*Acinonyxjubatus*) and Domestic Cat (*Felis silvestris f. catus*)." *Journal of Anatomy* 201, no. 3 (2002): 195–209.

Westgarth, Carrie, Robert M. Christley, and Hayley E. Christian. "How Might we Increase Physical Activity through Dog Walking?: A Comprehensive Review of Dog Walking Correlates." *International Journal of Behavioral Nutrition and Physical Activity* 11, art. 83 (2014).

Wong Kate. "Scrappy Pets." *Scientific American*, March 2013, 24.

CHAPTER 3: THE FAULT ISN'T IN OUR FOOD

Brand-Miller, Jennie, and Alan Barclay. "Declining Consumption of Added Sugars and Sugar-Sweetened Beverages in Australia: A Challenge for Obesity Prevention." *American Journal of Clinical Nutrition* 105, no. 4 (2017): 854–63.

DiNicolantonio, James J., Sean C. Lucan, and James H. O'Keefe. "The Evidence for Saturated Fat and for Sugar Related to Coronary Heart Disease." *Progress in Cardiovascular Diseases* 58, no. 5 (2016): 464–72.

Healy, Genevieve N., et al. "Objectively Measured Sedentary Time, Physical Activity, and Metabolic Risk." *Diabetes Care* 31, no. 2 (2008): 369–71.

Oliver, J. Eric. *Fat Politics: The Real Story Behind America's Obesity Epidemic*. Oxford: Oxford University Press, 2005.

Roth, Gregory A., et al. "Global, Regional, and National Burden of Cardiovascular Diseases for 10 Causes, 1990 to 2015." *Journal of the American College of Cardiology* 70, no. 1 (2017): 1–25.

Stanhope, Kimber L. "Sugar Consumption, Metabolic Disease and Obesity: The State of the Controversy." *Critical Reviews in Clinical Laboratory Sciences* 53, no. 1 (2016): 52–67.

Stuckler, David, Aaron Reeves, Rachel Loopstra, and Martin McKee. "Textual Analysis of Sugar Industry Influence on the World Health Organization's 2015 Sugars Intake Guideline." *Bulletin of the World Health Organization* 94 (2016): 566–73.

World Health Organization. "Guideline: Sugars Intake for Adults and Children." Geneva, Switzerland, 2015.

Zock, Peter L., Wendy A. Blom, Joyce A. Nettleton, and Gerard Hornstra. "Progressing Insights into the Role of Dietary Fats in the Prevention of Cardiovascular Disease." *Current Cardiology Reports* 18, no. 11 (2016): 111.

CHAPTER 4: MEATY MICE AND THE MEN AND WOMEN WHO OVER-FEED THEM

Ankeny, Rachel A. "Historiographic Reflections on Model Organisms: Or How the Mureaucracy May Be Limiting our Understanding of Contemporary Genetics and Genomics." *History and Philosophy of the Life Sciences* 32, no. 1 (2010): 91–104.

Baig, Ulfat, et al. "Foraging Theory and the Propensity to be Obese: An Alternative to Thrift." *Homo: internationale Zeitschrift fur die vergleichende Forschung am Menschen* 70, no. 3 (2019): 193–216.

Beans, Carolyn. "What Happens When Lab Animals Go Wild." *Proceedings of the National Academy of Sciences of the United States of America* 115, no. 13 (2018): 3196–99.

Bryda, Elizabeth C. "The Mighty Mouse: The Impact of Rodents on Advances in Biomedical Research." *Missouri Medicine* 110, no. 3 (2013): 207–11.

Byers, Kaylee. A., et al. "Rats about Town: A Systematic Review of Rat Movement in Urban Ecosystems." *Frontiers in Ecology and Evolution* 7, no. 13 (2019).

Carbone, Larry. Interview by author. June 2, 2021.

Even, Patrick C., et al. "Editorial: Are Rodent Models Fit for Investigation of Human Obesity and Related Diseases?" *Frontiers in Nutrition* 4, no. 58 (2017).

Flores-Opazo, Marcelo, Sean McGee, and Mark Hargreaves. "Exercise and GLUT4." *Exercise and Sport Sciences Reviews* 48, no. 3 (2020): 110–18.

Garner, Joseph P., et al. "Introducing Therioepistemology: The Study of How Knowledge Is Gained from Animal Research." *Lab Animal* 46, no. 4 (2017): 103–13.

Goodman, Justin, Alka Chandna, and Katherine Roe. "Trends in Animal Use at U.S. Research Facilities." *Journal of Medical Ethics* 41, no. 7 (2015): 567–69.

Goodpaster, Bret H., and Donna Wolf. "Skeletal Muscle Lipid Accumulation in Obesity, Insulin Resistance, and Type 2 Diabetes." *Pediatric Diabetes* 5, no. 4 (2004): 219–26.

Goodyear, Laurie J. Interview by author. May 26, 2021.

Goodyear, Laurie J., Michael F. Hirshman, and Edward S. Horton. "Exercise-Induced Translocation of Skeletal Muscle Glucose Transporters." *American Journal of Physiology* 261, no. 6 (1991): E795–99.

Hargreaves, Mark, and Lawrence L. Spriet. "Skeletal Muscle Energy Metabolism during Exercise." *Nature Metabolism* 2, no. 8 (2020): 817–28.

Kaur, Pali. Interview by author. October 15, 2021.

King, Aileen J. F. "The Use of Animal Models in Diabetes Research." *British Journal of Pharmacology* 166, no. 3 (2012): 877–94.

Koves, Timothy R., et al. "Mitochondrial Overload and Incomplete Fatty Acid Oxidation Contribute to Skeletal Muscle Insulin Resistance." *Cell Metabolism* 7, no. 1 (2008): 45–56.

Li, Yiran, et al. "Skeletal Intramyocellular Lipid Metabolism and Insulin Resistance." *Biophysics Reports* 1 (2015): 90–98.

Makowska, Johanna. Interview by author. June 7, 2021.

Martin, Bronwen, Sunggoan Ji, Stuart Maudsley, and Mark P. Mattson. "'Control' Laboratory Rodents Are Metabolically Morbid: Why It Matters." *Proceedings of the National Academy of Sciences* 107, no. 14 (2010): 6127–33.

Meijer, Johanna H. Interview by author. June 14, 2021.

Morales, Pablo Esteban, José Luis Bucarey, and Alejandra Espinosa. "Muscle Lipid Metabolism: Role of Lipid Droplets and Perilipins." *Journal of Diabetes Research* (2017): 1789395.

Park, Sung Sup, and Young-Kyo Seo. "Excess Accumulation of Lipid Impairs Insulin Sensitivity in Skeletal Muscle." *International Journal of Molecular Sciences* 21, no. 6 (2020).

Peggs, Kay. "Transgenic Animals, Biomedical Experiments, and 'Progress.'" *Journal of Animal Ethics* 3, no. 1 (Spring 2013): 41–56.

Pell, Richard W., and Lauren B. Allen. "Bringing Postnatural History into View." *American Scientist* 103, no. 3 (2015): 224–27.

Pell, Richard. Interview by author. June 22, 2021.

Rosenthal, Nadia. Interview by author. July 7, 2021.

Schock, Jaimie N. "Of Mice & Men." *American Society for Engineering Education's Prism* 22, no. 7-8 (2013): 34–37.

Stanford, Kristin I., and Laurie J. Goodyear. "Exercise and Type 2 Diabetes: Molecular Mechanisms Regulating Glucose Uptake in Skeletal Muscle." *Advances in Physiology Education* 38, no. 4 (2014): 308–14.

Sundberg, John P., and Paul N. Schofield. "Living Inside the Box: Environmental Effects on Mouse Models of Human Disease." *Disease Models & Mechanisms* 11, no. 10 (2018).

Tschöp, Matthias H., et al. "A Guide to Analysis of Mouse Energy Metabolism." *Nature Methods* 9, no. 1 (2011): 57–63.

Tunduguru, Ragadeepthi, and Debbie C. Thurmond. "Promoting Glucose Transporter-4 Vesicle Trafficking along Cytoskeletal Tracks: PAK-Ing Them Out." *Frontiers of Endocrinology* 8, no. 329 (2017).

Turcotte, Lorraine P., and Jonathan S. Fisher. "Skeletal Muscle Insulin Resistance: Roles of Fatty Acid Metabolism and Exercise." *Physical Therapy* 88, no. 11 (2008): 1279–96.

Wadman, Meredith. "Researchers Protest against Minimum Cage Sizes for Breeding Rodents." *Nature*, January 19, 2012.

Wanner, Mark. Interview by author. July 8, 2021.

Watt, Matthew J., and Andrew J. Hoy. "Lipid Metabolism in Skeletal Muscle: Generation of Adaptive and Maladaptive Intracellular Signals for Cellular

Function." *American Journal of Physiology Endocrinology and Metabolism* 302, no. 11 (2012): E1315–28.

Wojtaszewski Jorgen F. P., et al. "Exercise Modulates Postreceptor Insulin Signaling and Glucose Transport in Muscle-Specific Insulin Receptor Knockout Mice." *Journal of Clinical Investigation* 104, no. 9 (1999):1257–64.

Yeo, Wee Kian, et al. "Fat Adaptation in Well-Trained Athletes: Effects on Cell Metabolism." *Applied Physiology, Nutrition, and Metabolism* 36, no. 1 (2011): 12–22.

Zapata, Agustin, et al. "Microdialysis in Rodents." *Current Protocols in Neuroscience* (2009): unit 7.2.

CHAPTER 5: HOW FOOD FIGHTS HIJACKED OUR HEALTH

Barry, Vaughn W., et al. "Fitness vs. Fatness on All-Cause Mortality: A Meta-Analysis." *Progress In Cardiovascular Diseases* 56, no. 4 (2014): 382–90.

Blackburn, Henry. Interview by author. October 25, 2017; December 8, 2021; and December 21, 2021.

Bray, George. Interview by author. March 23, 2020.

Carlson, Susan A., et al. "Inadequate Physical Activity and Health Care Expenditures in the United States." *Progress in Cardiovascular Diseases* 57, no. 4 (2015): 315–23.

Church, Timothy S., et al. "Trends Over 5 decades in U.S. Occupation-Related Physical Activity and Their Associations with Obesity." *PloS One* 6, no. 5 (2011): e19657.

Duncan, Glen E. Interview by author. November 22, 2021.

Duncan, Glen E. "The 'Fit but Fat' Concept Revisited: Population-Based Estimates using NHANES." *International Journal of Behavioral Nutrition and Physical Activity* 7, art. 47 (2010).

Farrell, Steve. Interview by author. January 3, 2022.

Flegal, Katherine M. Interview by author. August 12, 2021.

Flegal, Katherine M. "The Obesity Wars and the Education of a Researcher: A Personal Account." *Progress in Cardiovascular Diseases* 67, no. 10 (2021): 75–79.

Flegal, Katherine M., Margaret D. Carroll, Cynthia L. Ogden, and Clifford L. Johnson. "Prevalence and Trends in Obesity among U.S. Adults, 1999–2000." *Journal of the American Medical Association* 288, no. 14 (2002): 1723–27.

Flegal, Katherine M., Margaret D. Carrol, and Robert J. Kuczmarski. "Overweight and Obesity in the United States: Prevalence and Trends, 1960–1994." *International Journal of Obesity* 22, no. 1 (1998): 39–47.

Flegal, Katherine M., Barry I. Graubard, David F. Williamson, and Mitchell H. Gail. "Excess Deaths Associated with Underweight, Overweight, and Obesity." *Journal of the American Medical Association* 293, no. 15 (2005):1861–67.

Flegal Katherine M., Barry I. Graubard, David F. Williamson, and Mitchell H. Gail. "Cause-Specific Excess Deaths Associated with Underweight, Overweight, and Obesity." *Journal of the American Medical Association JAMA* 298, no. 17 (2007): 2028–37.

Gaesser, Glenn A., and Siddhartha S. Angadi. "Obesity Treatment: Weight Loss versus Increasing Fitness and Physical Activity for Reducing Health Risks." *iScience* 24, no. 10 (2021): 102995.

Gaesser, Glenn A. Interview by author. October 12, 2021.

Global Burden of Disease, 2015 Obesity Collaborators. "Health Effects of Overweight and Obesity in 195 Countries over 25 Years." *New England Journal of Medicine* 377, no. 1 (2017): 13–27.

Hebert, James R., David B. Allison, Edward Archer, Carl J. Lavie, and Steven N. Blair. "Scientific Decision Making, Policy Decision, and the Obesity Pandemic." *Mayo Clinical Proceedings* 88, no. 6 (2013): P593–604.

Jacobs, David R., et al. "Cigarette Smoking and Mortality Risk: Twenty-Five-Year Follow-up of the Seven Countries Study." *Archives of Internal Medicine* 159, no. 7 (1999): 733–40.

Jensen, Michael D., et al. "2013 AHA/ACC/TOS Guideline for the Management of Overweight and Obesity in Adults." *Circulation* 129, no. 25, suppl. 2 (2014): S1–S45.

Keys, Ancel, et al. "Epidemiological Studies Related to Coronary Heart Disease: Characteristics of Men Aged 40-59 in Seven Countries." *Acta Medica Scandinavica* 460, suppl. (1967): 1–392.

Keys, Ancel, et al. "Physical Activity and the Diet in Populations Differing in Serum Cholesterol." *Journal of Clinical Investigation* 35, no. 10 (1956): 1173–81.

Kirkland, Anna. "The Environmental Account of Obesity: A Case for Feminist Skepticism." *Signs* 36, no. 2 (2011): 463–85.

"Obesity." *British Medical Journal* 2, no. 3901 (1935): 681–82.

Kosola, Jussi, et al. "Good Aerobic or Muscular Fitness Protects Overweight Men from Elevated Oxidized LDL." *Medicine & Science in Sports & Exercise* 44, no. 4 (April 1, 2012): 563–68.

Kramer, Caroline K., Bernard Zinman, and Ravi Retnakaran. "Are Metabolically Healthy Overweight and Obesity Benign Conditions? A Systemic Review and Meta Analysis." *Annals of Internal Medicine* 159, no. 11 (2013): 758–69.

Lee, Junga. "Influences of Cardiovascular Fitness and Body Fatness on the Risk of Metabolic Syndrome: A Systematic Review and Meta-Analysis." *American Journal of Health Promotion* 34, no. 7 (2020): 796–805.

Leon, Arthur. Interview by author. October 24, 2017.

López Coleman, Martha. Interview by author. November 12, 2021.

Mattson, Mark P. Interview by author. August 2, 2021.

Mitchell, Nia S., et al. "Obesity: Overview of an Epidemic." *Psychiatric Clinics of North America* 34, no. 4 (2011): 717–32.

Oktay, Ahmet Afşin, et al. "The Interaction of Cardiorespiratory Fitness with Obesity and the Obesity Paradox in Cardiovascular Disease." *Progress in Cardiovascular Diseases* 60, no. 1 (2017): 30–44.

Rea, Philip A., Peter Yin, and Ryan Zahalka. "Can Skinny Fat Beat Obesity?" *American Scientist* 102, no. 4 (2014): 272–79.

Rosen, Howard. "Is Obesity a Disease or a Behavior Abnormality? Did the AMA Get It Right?" *Missouri Medicine* 111, no. 2 (2014): 104–8.

Stokes, Andrew, and Samuel H. Preston. "How Dangerous Is Obesity? Issues in Measurement and Interpretation." *Population and Development Review* 42, no. 4 (2016): 595–614.

Strings, Sabrina. "Obese Black Women as 'Social Dead Weight': Reinventing the 'Diseased Black Woman.'" *Signs* 41, no. 1 (Autumn 2015): 107–30.

Swidey, Neil. "Walter Willett's Food Fight." *Boston Globe*, July 28, 2013.

Tracy, Sarah. Interview by author. December 13, 2017.

Ulijaszek, Stanley J., and Hayley Lofink. "Obesity in Biocultural Perspective." *Annual Review of Anthropology* 35 (2006): 337–60.

Yacamán-Méndez, Diego, et al. "Author Correction: Life-Course Trajectories of Weight and Their Impact on the Incidence of Type 2 Diabetes." *Scientific Reports* 11, no. 1 (2021): 18602.

CHAPTER 6: TREADMILL-TROTTING PIGS

Addison, Odessa, Robin L. Marcus, Paul C. LaStayo, and Alice S. Ryan. "Intermuscular Fat: A Review of the Consequences and Causes." *International Journal of Endocrinology* (2014): 309570.

Altmann, Stuart A. "Fallback Foods, Eclectic Omnivores, and the Packaging Problem." *American Journal of Physical Anthropology* 140, no. 4 (2009): 615–29.

Antunes, Barbara de Moura Mello, et al. "Exercise Intensity and Physical Fitness Modulate Lipoproteins Profile during Acute Aerobic Exercise Session." *Scientific Reports* 10, no. 1 (2020): 4160.

Armamento-Villareal, Reina, Nicola Napoli, Debra Waters, and Villareal Dennis. "Fat, Muscle, and Bone Interactions in Obesity and the Metabolic Syndrome." *International Journal of Endocrinology* (2014): 247076.

Azevedo, Paula S., et al. "Cardiac Remodeling: Concepts, Clinical Impact, Pathophysiological Mechanisms and Pharmacologic Treatment." *Arquivos brasileiros de cardiologia* 106, no. 1 (2016): 62–69.

Bassuk Shari S., and Manson JoAnn E. "Epidemiological Evidence for the Role of Physical Activity in Reducing Risk of Type 2 Diabetes and Cardiovascular Disease." *Journal of Applied Physiology* 99, no. 3 (2005): 1193–204.

Bjørndal, Bodil, et al. "Different Adipose Depots: Their Role in the Development of Metabolic Syndrome and Mitochondrial Response to Hypolipidemic Agents." *Journal of Obesity* no. 490650 (2011).

Brisbin, Jr., I. Lehr, and Michael S. Sturek. "The Pigs of Ossabaw Island: A Case Study of the Application of Long-Term Data in Management Plan Development." In *Wild Pigs: Biology, Damage, Control Techniques and Management*-SRNL-RP-2009-00869, edited by John Mayer and I. Lehr Brisbin Jr., 365–78. Aiken, SC: Savannah River National Laboratory, 2009.

Brisbin, Jr., I. Lehr. Interview by author. September 29, 2018.

Bruning, Rebecca S., and Michael Sturek. "Benefits of Exercise Training on Coronary Blood Flow in Coronary Artery Disease Patients." *Progress in Cardiovascular Diseases* 57, no. 5 (2015): 443–53.

Carley, Andrew N., Heinrich Taegtmeyer, and E. Douglas Lewandowski. "Matrix Revisited: Mechanisms Linking Energy Substrate Metabolism to the Function of the Heart." *Circulation Research* 114, no. 4 (2014): 717–29.

Dawson, Harry. "Comparative Nutrigenomics of the Pig, Mouse and Human; Linking Phenotype to Genotype for Improved Models of Human and Swine Nutrition." *Journal of Animal Science* 96, no. 3 (2018): 292.

Day, Kara. Interview by author. September 27, 2018.

Dostálová, Anne, Alena Svitáková, Daniel Bureš, Libor Vališ, and Zdeněk Volek. "Effect of an Outdoor Access System on the Growth Performance, Carcass Characteristics, and *Longissimus lumborum* Muscle Meat Quality of the Prestice Black-Pied Pig Breed." *Animals: An Open Access Journal from MDPI* 10, no. 8 (2020): 1244.

Dyson Melissa C., et al. "Components of Metabolic Syndrome and Coronary Artery Disease in Female Ossabaw Swine Fed Excess Atherogenic Diet." *Comparative Medicine* 56, no. 1 (2006): 35–45.

Edwards, Jason N., et al. "Exercise Training Decreases Store-Operated Ca2+ Entry Associated with Metabolic Syndrome and Coronary Atherosclerosis." *Cardiovascular Research* 85, no. 3 (2010): 631–40.

Gerstein, Hertzel C., and Laura Waltman. "Why Don't Pigs Get Diabetes? Explanations for Variations in Diabetes Susceptibility in Human Populations Living in a Diabetogenic Environment." *Canadian Medical Association Journal* 174, no. 1 (2006): 25-6.

Hardie, Ann. "The Old Lady of Ossabaw." *Atlanta*, March 1, 2011.

Hargreaves, Mark, and Lawrence L. Spriet. "Skeletal Muscle Energy Metabolism during Exercise." *Nature Metabolism* 2, no. 9 (2020): 817–28.

Hausman, Gary J., et al. "Intermuscular and Intramuscular Adipose Tissues: Bad vs. Good Adipose Tissues." *Adipocyte* 3, no. 4 (2014): 242–55.

Hawley, John A., and Jill J. Leckey. "Carbohydrate Dependence During Prolonged, Intense Endurance Exercise." *Sports Medicine* 45, no. 1 (2015): S5–12.

Karasov, William H., and Angela E. Douglas. "Comparative Digestive Physiology." *Comprehensive Physiology* 3, no. 2 (2013): 741–83.

Magkos, Faidon, et al. "Free Fatty Acid Kinetics in the Late Phase of Postexercise Recovery: Importance of Resting Fatty Acid Metabolism and Exercise-Induced Energy Deficit." *Metabolism: Clinical and Experimental* 58, no. 9 (2009): 1248–55.

Nielsen, Kirstine L., et al. "Similar Metabolic Responses in Pigs and Humans to Breads with Different Contents and Compositions of Dietary Fibers: A Metabolomics Study." *American Journal of Clinical Nutrition* 99, no. 4 (2014): 941–9.

Ruiz-Ramie, Jonathan J., Jacob L. Barber, and Mark A. Sarzynski. "Effects of Exercise on HDL Functionality." *Current Opinion in Lipidology* 30, no. 1 (2019): 16–23.

Penney, Veronica. "Eleanor Torrey West, Preserver of Her Inherited Island, Dies at 108." *New York Times*, January 28, 2021.

Shuster, Anatoly, Michael Patlas, Jehonathan H. Pinthus, and Marina Mourtzakis. "The Clinical Importance of Visceral Adiposity: A Critical Review of Methods for Visceral Adipose Tissue Analysis." *British Journal of Radiology* 85, no. 1009 (2012): 1–10.

Stanley, William C., Fabio A. Recchia, and Gary D. Lopaschuk. "Myocardial Substrate Metabolism in the Normal and Failing Heart." *Physiological Reviews* 85, no. 3 (2005): 1093–129.

"Study Offers Another Incentive for Flat Abs." *All Things Considered*, National Public Radio, November 12, 2008.

Sturek, Michael. "Ca2+ Regulatory Mechanisms of Exercise Protection against Coronary Artery Disease in Metabolic Syndrome and Diabetes." *Journal of Applied Physiology* 111, no. 2 (2011): 573–86.

Sturek, Michael. Interview by author. October 4, 2018, and November 15, 2018.

Trask, Aaron J., et al. "Dynamic Micro- and Macrovascular Remodeling in Coronary Circulation of Obese Ossabaw Pigs with Metabolic Syndrome." *Journal of Applied Physiology* 113, no. 7 (2012): 1128–40.

Turcotte, Lorraine P., and Jonathan S. Fisher. "Skeletal Muscle Insulin Resistance: Roles of Fatty Acid Metabolism and Exercise." *Physical Therapy* 88, no. 11 (2008): 1279–96.

US Department of the Interior, National Park Service. "Ossabaw Island: National Register of Historic Places Registration Form." OMB no. 1024-0018, Washington, DC, March 25, 1996.

Välimäki, Iiro A., et al. "Strenuous Physical Exercise Accelerates the Lipid Peroxide Clearing Transport by HDL." *European Journal of Applied Physiology* 116, no. 9 (2016): 1683–91.

Vargas-Ortiz, Katya, et al. "Exercise and Sirtuins: A Way to Mitochondrial Health in Skeletal Muscle." *International Journal of Molecular Sciences* 20, no. 11 (2019): 2717.

Wigernæs, Ine, Arne T. Høstmark, Sigmund B. Strømme, Peter Kierulf, and Kåre Birkeland. "Active Recovery and Post-Exercise White Blood Cell Count, Free Fatty Acids, and Hormones in Endurance Athletes." *European Journal of Applied Physiology* 84, no. 4 (2001): 358–66.

Wright, Chris. "The Battle for America's Miracle Pig." *Gear Patrol*, October 31, 2016.

Zacharewicz, Evelyn, Matthijs K. C. Hesselink, and Patrick Schrauwen. "Exercise Counteracts Lipotoxicity by Improving Lipid Turnover and Lipid Droplet Quality." *Journal of Internal Medicine* 284, no. 5 (2018): 505–18.

Zhang, Yun, Joanna Yang, Wei Hou, and Chrisa Arcan. "Obesity Trends and Associations with Types of Physical Activity and Sedentary Behavior in U.S. Adults: National Health and Nutrition Examination Survey, 2007–2016." *Obesity* 29, no. 1 (2021): 24–50.

Ziegler, Amanda, Liara Gonzalez, and Anthony Blikslager. "Large Animal Models: The Key to Translational Discovery in Digestive Disease Research." *Cellular and Molecular Gastroenterology and Hepatology* 2, no. 6 (2016): 716–24.

CHAPTER 7: BACKSTROKE-SWIMMING ROUNDWORMS

Aagaard-Hansen, Jens, and Claire Lise Chaignat. "Neglected Tropical Diseases: Equity and Social Determinants." In *Equity, Social Determinants and Public Health Programmes*, edited by Erik Blas and Anand Sivasankara Kurup, 135–57. Geneva: World Health Organization, 2010.

Auld, Stewart K. J. R., and Matthew C. Tinsley. "The Evolutionary Ecology of Complex Lifecycle Parasites: Linking Phenomena with Mechanisms." *Heredity* 114, no. 2 (2015): 125–32.

Bannister, David. "Public Health and Its Contexts in Northern Ghana, 1900–2000." PhD diss., SOAS University of London, 2017.

Chaudhari, Snehal N., and Edward T. Kipreos. "Increased Mitochondrial Fusion Allows the Survival of Older Animals in Diverse *C. elegans* Longevity Pathways." *Nature Communications* 8, art. 182 (2017).

Chuang, Han Sheng, Wan-Jung Kuo, Chia-Lin Lee, I-Hua Chu, and Chang-Shi Chen. "Exercise in an Electrotactic Flow Chamber Ameliorates Age-Related Degeneration in *Caenorhabditis elegans*." *Scientific Reports* 6 (2016): 28064.

Cook, Gordon Charles. "Early History of Clinical Tropical Medicine in London." *Journal of the Royal Society of Medicine* 83 (1990): 38–41.

Correale, Jorge, and Mauricio F. Farez. "The Impact of Environmental Infections (Parasites) on MS Activity." *Multiple Sclerosis Journal* 17, no. 10 (2011): 1162–69.

Correale, Jorge, Mariano Marrodan, and Edgar Carnero Contentti. "Interleukin-35 Is a Critical Regulator of Immunity during Helminth Infections Associated with Multiple Sclerosis." *Immunology* 164, no. 3 (2021): 569–86.

Croese, John, Soraya T. Gaze, and Alex Loukas. "Changed Gluten Immunity in Celiac Disease by *Necator Americanus* Provides New Insights into Autoimmunity." *International Journal for Parasitology* 43, no. 3-4 (2013): 275–82.

Cross, John H. "Enteric Nematodes of Humans." In *Medical Microbiology, 4th ed.*, edited by Samuel Baron, chapter 90. Galveston: University of Texas Medical Branch at Galveston, 1996.

Cox, Francis E. G. "History of Human Parasitology." *Clinical Microbiology Reviews* 15, no. 4 (2002): 595–612.

Etya'ale, Daniel. "Vision 2020: Update on Onchocerciasis." *Community Eye Health* 14, no. 38 (2001): 19–21.

Fleming, John O., and Thomas D. Cook. "Multiple Sclerosis and the Hygiene Hypothesis." *Neurology* 67, no. 11 (2006): 2085-86.

Frézal, Lise and Marie-Anne Félix. "The Natural History of Model Organisms: *C. elegans* outside the Petri Dish." *eLife Sciences Publications Limited* 4 (2015): e05849.

Frias, Liesbeth, et al. "A Pinworm's Tale: The Evolutionary History of *Lemuricola (Protenterobius) nycticebi*." *International Journal of Parasitology: Parasites and Wildlife* 8 (2019): 25–32.

Giannelli, Alessio, Cinzia Cantacessi, Vito Colella, Filipe Dantas-Torres, and Domenico Otranto. "Gastropod-Borne Helminths: A Look at the Snail-Parasite Interplay." *Trends in Parasitology* 32, no. 3 (2016): 255–64.

Gustavsen, Ken, Adrian Hopkins, and Mauricio Sauerbrey. "Onchocerciasis in the Americas: From Arrival to (Near) Elimination." *Parasites & Vectors* 4, no. 1, art. 205 (2011).

Haque, Rashidul. "Human Intestinal Parasites." *Journal of Health, Population, and Nutrition* 25, no. 4 (2007): 387–91.

Hartman, Jessica H., et al. "Swimming Exercise and Transient Food Deprivation in *Caenorhabditis elegans* Promote Mitochondrial Maintenance and Protect Against Chemical-Induced Mitotoxicity." *Scientific Reports* 8, no. 1, art. 8359 (2018).

Hartman, Jessica H. Interview by author. September 30, 2021.

Hirsch, Lioba. "The LSHTM and Colonialism: History and Legacy-Draft Protocol." Research project, Centre for History in Public Health, London, January 2020.

Hotez, Peter J., et al. "Helminth Infections: The Great Neglected Tropical Diseases." *Journal of Clinical Investigation* 118, no. 4 (2008): 1311–21.

Houweling, Tanja A. J., et al. "Socioeconomic Inequalities in Neglected Tropical Diseases: A Systematic Review." *PLoS Neglected Tropical Diseases* 10, no. 5 (2016): e0004546.

Keating, Conrad. "Ken Warren and the Rockefeller Foundation's Great Neglected Diseases Network, 1978–1988: The Transformation of Tropical and Global Medicine." *Molecular Medicine* 20, suppl. 1 (2014): S24–S30.

Laranjeiro, Ricardo, et al. "Swim Exercise in *Caenorhabditis elegans* Extends Neuromuscular and Gut Healthspan, Enhances Learning Ability, and Protects against Neurodegeneration." *PNAS* 116, no. 47 (2019): 23829–39.

Laranjeiro, Ricardo. Interview by author. September 21, 2021.

Proceedings of the National Academy of Sciences 116, no. 47 (2019): 23829–39.

Midha, Ankur, et al. "The Intestinal Roundworm *Ascaris suum* Releases Antimicrobial Factors Which Interfere with Bacterial Growth and Biofilm Formation." *Frontiers in Cellular and Infection Microbiology* 8, no. 271 (2018).

Montresor, Antonio. Interview by author. October 7, 2021.

Molyneux, David H., Anarfi Asamoa-Bah, Alan Fenwick, Lorenzo Savioli, and Peter Hotez. "The History of the Neglected Tropical Disease Movement." *Transactions of the Royal Society of Tropical Medicine and Hygiene* 115, no. 2 (2021): 169–75.

Ostkamp, Patrick, et al. "Sunlight Exposure Exerts Immunomodulatory Effects to Reduce Multiple Sclerosis Severity." *Proceedings of the National Academy of Sciences* 118, no. 1 (2021): e2018457118.

Padmanabhan, Venkat, et al. "Locomotion of *C. elegans*: A Piecewise-Harmonic Curvature Representation of Nematode Behavior." *PLoS One* 7, no 7 (2012): e40121.

Paige, Sarah B., et al. "Combining Footwear with Public Health Iconography to Prevent Soil-Transmitted Helminth Infections." *American Journal of Tropical Medicine and Hygiene* 96, no. 1 (2017): 205–13.

Reece, Sarah E., Kimberley F. Prior, and Nicole Mideo. "The Life and Times of Parasites: Rhythms in Strategies for Within-host Survival and Between-Host Transmission." *Journal of Biological Rhythms* 32, no. 6 (2017): 516–33.

Reinhard, Karl J., Richard H. Helvy, and Glenn A. Anderson. "Helminth Remains from Prehistoric Indian Coprolites on the Colorado Plateau." *Journal of Parasitology* 73, no. 3 (1987): 630–39.

Shahvisi, Arianne. Interview by author. October 11, 2021.

Shahvisi, Arianne. "Tropicality and Abjection: What Do We Really Mean by 'Neglected Tropical Diseases'?" *Developing World Bioethics* 19, no. 4 (2019): 224–34.

Smallwood, Taylor B., et al. "Helminth Immunomodulation in Autoimmune Disease." *Frontiers in Immunology* 8, no. 453 (2017).

Tanasescu, Radu, and Cris S. Constantinescu. "Helminth Therapy for MS." *Current Topics in Behavioral Neurosciences* 26 (2015): 195–220.

Tomczyk, Sara, et al. "Association between Footwear Use and Neglected Tropical Diseases: A Systematic Review and Meta-Analysis." *PLoS Neglected Tropical Diseases* 8, no. 11 (2014): e3285.

van den Hoogen, Johan, et al. "Soil Nematode Abundance and Functional Group Composition at a Global Scale." *Nature*, July 24, 2019, 194–8.

Wakelin Derek. "Helminths: Pathogenesis and Defenses." In *Medical Microbiology, 4th ed.*, edited by Samuel Baron, chapter 87. Galveston: University of Texas Medical Branch at Galveston, 1996.

Wegayehu, Teklu, Tsegaye Tsalla, Belete Seifu, and Takele Teklu. "Prevalence of Intestinal Parasitic Infections among Highland and Lowland Dwellers in Gamo Area, South Ethiopia." *BMC Public Health* 13, no. 151 (2013).

Wendt, Sebastian, et al. "The Diagnosis and Treatment of Pinworm Infection." *Deutsches Arzteblatt International* 116, no. 13 (2019): 213–19.

Xuting, Jin, et al. "Global Burden of Upper Respiratory Infections in 204 Countries and Territories, from 1990 to 2019." *Lancet, eClinical Medicine* 37, no. 100986 (2021).

Zarowiecki, Magdalena, and Matt Berriman. "What Helminth Genomes Have Taught Us about Parasite Evolution." *Parasitology* 142, no. 1 (2015): S85–97.

CHAPTER 8: THE MAN VERSUS HORSE MARATHON

Ahmetov, Ildus I., and Olga N. Fedotovskaya. "Current Progress in Sports Genomics." *Advances in Clinical Chemistry* 70 (2015): 247–314.

Alshak, Mark N., and Joe M. Das. *Neuroanatomy, Sympathetic Nervous System.* Treasure Island, FL: StatPearls Publishing, 2021.

Anderson, Ethan J., Hanae Yamazaki, and P. Darrell Neufer. "Induction of Endogenous Uncoupling Protein 3 Suppresses Mitochondrial Oxidant Emission during Fatty Acid-supported Respiration." *Journal of Biological Chemistry* 282, no. 43 (2007): 31257–66.

Angoules, Antonios G., Anna Christakou, Haridimos Tsibidakis, Georgios A. Angoules, and Stylianos Kapetanakis. "Horse–Related Spine and Spinal Cord Injuries." *Clinical Sciences Research and Reports* 2, (2019): 1-7-7-7.

Baker, Lindsay B. "Physiology of Sweat Gland Function: The roles of Sweating and Sweat Composition in Human Health." *Temperature* 6, no. 3 (2019): 211–59.

Baker, Lindsay B. "Sweating Rate and Sweat Sodium Concentration in Athletes: A Review of Methodology and Intra/Interindividual Variability." *Sports Medicine* 47, no. 1 (2017): 111–28.

Barnes, Kelly A., et al. "Normative Data for Sweating Rate, Sweat Sodium Concentration, and Sweat Sodium Loss in Athletes: An Update and Analysis by Sport." *Journal of Sports Sciences* 37, no. 20 (2019): 2356–66.

Barrett, Ron. Interview by author. July 13, 2021.

Bollinger, Lena, Alexander Bartel, Alina Küper, Corinna Weber, and Heidrun Gehlen. "Age and Hydration of Competing Horses Influence the Outcome of Elite 160 km Endurance Rides." *Frontiers in Veterinary Science* 8, no. 668650 (2021).

Bovell, Douglas L. "The Evolution of Eccrine Sweat Gland Research Towards Developing a Model for Human Sweat Gland Function." *Experimental Dermatology* 27, no. 5 (2018): 544–50.

Bouillaud, Frédéric, Marie-Clotilde Alves-Guerra, and Daniel Ricquier. "UCPs, at the Interface between Bioenergetics and Metabolism." *Biochimica et biophysica acta* 1863, no. 10 (2016): 2443–56.

Buchmann, Sylvia J., Ana Isabel Penzlin, Marie Luise Kubasch, Ben Min-Woo Illigens, and Timo Siepmann. "Assessment of Sudomotor Function." *Clinical Autonomic Research: Official Journal of the Clinical Autonomic Research Society* 29, no. 1 (2019): 41–53.

Chen, Yi-Lang, Wen-Hui Kuan, and Chao-Lin Liu. "Comparative Study of the Composition of Sweat from Eccrine and Apocrine Sweat Glands during Exercise and in Heat." *International Journal of Environmental Research and Public Health* 17, no. 10 (2020): 3377.

Collin, Yvette Running Horse. "The Relationship between the Indigenous Peoples of the Americas and the Horse: Deconstructing a Eurocentric Myth." PhD diss., University of Alaska Fairbanks, 2017.

Cortassa, Sonia, Miguel A. Aon, and Steven J. Sollott. "Control and Regulation of Substrate Selection in Cytoplasmic and Mitochondrial Catabolic Networks. A Systems Biology Analysis." *Frontiers in Physiology* 10, no. 201 (2019).

Coury, Nick. Interview by author. August 4, 2021.

Cowles, Jr., R. Reynolds. "Emergency Services at Steeplechase and Cross-Country Hunter Events." *American Association of Equine Practitioners Proceedings* 54 (2008): 153–56.

Dao, Christine Ky Linh. "The Underlying Mechanisms of UCP-3 Dependent Thermogenesis in Skeletal Muscle." PhD diss., University of Texas at Austin, 2015.

Davis, Michael S., and Montana R. Barrett. "Effect of Conditioning and Physiological Hyperthermia on Canine Skeletal Muscle Mitochondrial Oxygen Consumption." *Journal of Applied Physiology* 130, no. 5 (2021): 1317–25.

Demine, Stéphane, Patricia Renard, and Thierry Arnould. "Mitochondrial Uncoupling: A Key Controller of Biological Processes in Physiology and Diseases." *Cells* 8, no. 8 (2019): 795.

Donnally, Eddie, Rev. "Paraplegic Former Jockey Anne Von Rosen: 'I Will Walk Again.'" Paulick Report, January 23, 2015.

Forbes, Chris. "Anne Von Rosen." Femalejockeys.com. No date.

Gardiner, Virginia. Interview by author. February 28, 2022.

Gilbert, Matt Sakiestewa. *Hopi Runners: Crossing the Terrain between Indian and American*. Lawrence: University Press of Kansas, 2018.

Gilbert, Matt Sakiestewa. Interview by author. August 12, 2021.

Hamill, Rich. Interview by author. August 20, 2021.

Harper, Mary-Ellen. Interview by author. September 30, 2021.

Houser, Bradley Scott. Interview by author. August 11, 2021.

Huertas, Jesus R., Rafael A. Casuso, Pablo Hernansanz Agustín, and Sara Cogliati. "Stay Fit, Stay Young: Mitochondria in Movement: The Role of Exercise in the New Mitochondrial Paradigm." *Oxidative Medicine and Cellular Longevity* (2019): 7058350.

Illigens, Ben M. W., and Christopher H. Gibbons. "Sweat testing to evaluate autonomic function." *Clinical Autonomic Research: Official Journal of the Clinical Autonomic Research Society* 19, no. 2 (2009): 79–87.

Ironside, Marianne. Interview by author. August 23, 2021.

Jablonski, Nina G. "The Naked Truth: Why Humans Have No Fur." *Scientific American* 302, no. 2 (2010): 42–9.

Jiang, Ning, et al. "Upregulation of Uncoupling Protein-3 in Skeletal Muscle during Exercise: A Potential Antioxidant Function." *Free Radical Biology & Medicine* 46, no. 2 (2009): 138–45.

Jones-Wilkins, Andy. "Rest in Peace: Dennis Poolheco." Irunfar.com, June 12, 2015.

Kazamel, Mohamed. Interview by author. August 19, 2021.

Le Moyec, Laurence, et al. "A First Step Toward Unraveling the Energy Metabolism in Endurance Horses: Comparison of Plasma Nuclear Magnetic Resonance Metabolomic Profiles Before and After Different Endurance Race Distances." *Frontiers in Molecular Biosciences* 6, no. 45 (2019).

Lieberman, Daniel E., and Dennis M. Bramble. "The Evolution of Marathon Running Capabilities in Humans." *Sports Medicine* 37, no. 4-5 (2007): 288–90.

Lieberman, Daniel E. Interview by the author. December 15, 2020.

Marlin, David. Interview by author. September 16, 2021.

Mrakic-Sposta, Simona, et al. "Training Effects on ROS Production Determined by Electron Paramagnetic Resonance in Master Swimmers." *Oxidative Medicine and Cellular Longevity* (2015): 804794.

Neufer, P. Darrell. "The Bioenergetics of Exercise." Cold Spring Harbor Perspectives in Medicine 8, no. 5 (2018): a029678.

Nowinski, Sara M., et al. "Mitochondrial Fatty Acid Synthesis Coordinates Oxidative Metabolism in Mammalian Mitochondria." *eLife* 9 (2020): e58041.

Pablos, Edgar, and Judith Cummings, directors. *Long Distance Messenger: Dennis Poolheco.* Los Angeles: Tribesmen Pictures, 2016.

Pérez-Matos, Maria Camila, Martha Catalina Morales-Alvarez, and Carlos O. Mendivil. "Lipids: A Suitable Therapeutic Target in Diabetic Neuropathy?" *Journal of Diabetes Research* (2017): 6943851.

Periasamy, Muthu, Jose Luis Herrera, and Felipe C. G. Reis. "Skeletal Muscle Thermogenesis and Its Role in Whole Body Energy Metabolism." *Diabetes & Metabolism Journal* 41, no. 5 (2017): 327–36.

Poburko, Damon, and Nicolas Demaurex. "Regulation of the Mitochondrial Proton Gradient by Cytosolic Ca^2 Signals." *Pflugers Archiv European Journal of Physiology* 464, no. 1 (2012): 19–26.

Pohl, Elena E., Anne Rupprecht, Gabriel Macher, and Karolina E. Hilse. "Important Trends in UCP3 Investigation." *Frontiers in Physiology* 10, no. 470 (2019).

Porter, Alan M. W. "Why Do We Have Apocrine and Sebaceous Glands?" *Journal of the Royal Society of Medicine* 94, no. 5 (2001): 236–7.

Powers, Scott K., and Malcolm J. Jackson. "Exercise-Induced Oxidative Stress: Cellular Mechanisms and Impact on Muscle Force Production." *Physiological Reviews* 88, no. 4 (2008): 1243–76.

Raymond, Colin, Tom Matthews, and Radley M. Horton. "The Emergence of Heat and Humidity too Severe for Human Tolerance." *Science Advances* 6, no. 19 (2020): eaaw1838.

Riley, Christopher L., et al. "The Complementary and Divergent Roles of Uncoupling Proteins 1 and 3 in Thermoregulation." *Journal of Physiology* 594, no. 24 (2016): 7455–64.

Riley, Christopher L. Interview by author. August 30, 2021.

Robert, Céline, et al. "Hydration and Electrolyte Balance in Horses during an Endurance Season." *Equine Veterinary Journal* suppl. 38 (2010): 98–104.

Rousset, Sophie et al. "The Biology of Mitochondrial Uncoupling Proteins." *Diabetes* 53, suppl. 1 (2004): S130–35.

Schrauwen, Patrick, and Matthijs Hesselink. "Uncoupling Protein 3 and Physical Activity: The Role of Uncoupling Protein 3 in Energy Metabolism Revisited." *Proceedings of the Nutrition Society* 62, no. 3 (2003): 635–43.

Shibasaki, Manabu, and Craig G. Crandall. "Mechanisms and Controllers of Eccrine Sweating in Humans." *Frontiers in Bioscience*, scholar edition 2 (2010): 685–96.

Schicho, Andreas, Dominik Einwag, Alexander Eickhoff, Peter H. Richter, and Christoph Riepl. "Verletzungsfolgen nach Wirbelsäulenfrakturen im Reitsport" [Impact of Spinal Fractures in Horseback Riding]. *Sportverletz Sportschaden* 29, no. 4 (2015): 231–5.

Scholpa, Natalie E., and Rick G. Schnellmann. "Mitochondrial-Based Therapeutics for the Treatment of Spinal Cord Injury: Mitochondrial Biogenesis as a Potential Pharmacological Target." *Journal of Pharmacology and Experimental Therapeutics* 363, no. 3 (2017): 303–13.

Steinbacher, Peter, and Peter Eckl. "Impact of Oxidative Stress on Exercising Skeletal Muscle." *Biomolecules* 5, no. 2 (2015): 356–77.

Von Rosen, Anne. Interview by author. August 20, 2021.

Wikström, Mårten, and Roger Springett. "Thermodynamic Efficiency, Reversibility, and Degree of Coupling in Energy Conservation by the Mitochondrial Respiratory Chain." *Communications Biology* 3, no. 1 (2020): 451.

"Were Horses in Native Culture before the Settlers Came? New Study Says Yes." *Navajo-Hopi Observer*, July 23, 2019.

Zhao, Ru-Zhou, Shuai Jiang, Lin Zhang, and Zhi-Bin Yu. "Mitochondrial Electron Transport Chain, ROS Generation and Uncoupling (Review)." *International Journal of Molecular Medicine* 44, no. 1 (2019): 3–15.

CHAPTER 9: BATS, BABIES, AND IMMUNITY

Bharati, Jaya, et al. "Expression Dynamics of HSP70 during Chronic Heat Stress in Tharparkar Cattle." *International Journal of Biometeorology* 61, no. 6 (2017): 1017–27.

Bjornevik, Kjetil, et al. "Longitudinal Analysis Reveals High Prevalence of Epstein-Barr Virus Associated with Multiple Sclerosis." *Science* 375, no. 6578 (2022): 296–301.

Canals, Mauricio L., Jose Iriarte-Diaz, and Bruno Grossi. "Biomechanical, Respiratory and Cardiovascular Adaptations of Bats and the Case of the Small Community of Bats in Chile." In *Biomechanics in Applications*, edited by Vaclav Klika, 299-322. London: InTechOpen Limited, 2011.

Chionh, Yok Teng, et al. "High Basal Heat-Shock Protein Expression in Bats Confers Resistance to Cellular Heat/Oxidative Stress." *Cell Stress Chaperones* 24, no. 4 (2019): 835–49.

Ekblom-Bak, Elin, et al. "Cardiorespiratory Fitness and Lifestyle on Severe COVID-19 Risk in 279,455 Adults: A Case Control Study." *International Journal of Behavioral Nutrition and Physical Activity* 18, no. 1, art. 135 (2021).

Ely, Brett R., Zachary S. Clayton, Carrie E. McCurdy, Joshua Pfeiffer, and Christopher T. Minson. "Meta-Inflammation and Cardiometabolic Disease in Obesity: Can Heat Therapy Help?" *Temperature* 5, no. 1 (2017): 9–21.

Gentile, Antonietta, et al. "Immunomodulatory Effects of Exercise in Experimental Multiple Sclerosis." *Frontiers in Immunology* 10, no. 2197 (2019).

Göbel, Kerstin, Tobias Ruck, and Sven G. Meuth. "Cytokine Signaling in Multiple Sclerosis: Lost in Translation." *Multiple Sclerosis Journal* 24, no. 4 (2018): 432–39.

Guglielmo, Christopher G. "Move That Fatty Acid: Fuel Selection and Transport in Migratory Birds and Bats." *Integrative and Comparative Biology* 50, no. 3 (2010): 336–45.

Dangi, Satyaveer Singh, et al. "Expression Profile of HSP Genes during Different Seasons in Goats (*Capra hircus*)." *Tropical Animal Health and Production* 44, no. 8 (2012): 1905–12.

Henstridge, Darren C., Mark A. Febbraio, and Mark Hargreaves. "Heat Shock Proteins and Exercise Adaptations: Our Knowledge Thus Far and the Road Still Ahead." *Journal of Applied Physiology* 120, no. 6 (2016): 683–91.

Irving, Aaron Trent. Interview by author. May 4, 2020.

Gibson, Oliver R., James A. Tuttle, Peter W. Watt, Neil S. Maxwell, and Lee Taylor. "Hsp72 and Hsp90α mRNA transcription Is Characterised by Large, Sustained Changes in Core Temperature during Heat Acclimation." *Cell Stress Chaperones* 21, no. 6 (2016): 1021–35.

Khandia, Rekha, Ashok K. Munjal, Hafiz M. Nn Iqbal, and Kuldeep Dhama. "Heat Shock Proteins: Therapeutic Perspectives in Inflammatory Disorders." *Recent Patents on Inflammation & Allergy Drug Discovery* 10, no. 2 (2017): 94–104.

Krause, Mauricio, Fernando Gerchman, and Rogério Friedman. "Coronavirus Infection (SARS-CoV-2) in Obesity and Diabetes Comorbidities: Is Heat Shock Response Determinant for the Disease Complications?" *Diabetology & Metabolic Syndrome* 12, art. 63 (2020).

Libbey, Jane E., and Robert S. Fujinami. "Potential triggers of MS." *Molecular Basis of Multiple Sclerosis* 51 (2010): 21–42.

Mandl, Judith N., Caitlin Schneider, David S. Schneider, and Michelle L. Baker. "Going to Bat(s) for Studies of Disease Tolerance." *Frontiers in Immunology* 9, art. 2112 (2018).

Mansilla, Maria José, Xavier Montalban, and Carmen Espejo. "Heat Shock Protein 70: Roles in Multiple Sclerosis." *Molecular Medicine* 18, no. 1 (2012): 1018–28.

McCracken, Gary. Interview by author. November 5, 2020.

McCool, Addison. Interview by author. August 25, 2020.

Medellin, Rodrigo A., et al. "Follow Me: Foraging Distances of *Leptonycteris yerbabuenae* (Chiroptera: Phyllostomidae) in Sonora Determined by Fluorescent Powder." *Journal of Mammalogy* 9, no. 2 (2018): 306–11.

Meyer, Christoph F. J., Moritz Weinbeer, and Elisabeth K. V. Kalko. "Home-Range Size and Spacing Patterns of *Macrophyllum macrophyllum* (Phyllostomidae) Foraging over Water." *Journal of Mammalogy* 86, no. 3 (2005): 587–98.

Gentile, Antonietta, et al. "Immunomodulatory Effects of Exercise in Experimental Multiple Sclerosis." *Frontiers in Immunology* 10, art. 2197 (2019).

Gilden, Donald H. "Infectious Causes of Multiple Sclerosis." *Lancet: Neurology* 4, no. 3 (2005): 195–202.

Heck, Thiago Gomes, Mirna Stela Ludwig, Matias Nunes Frizzo, Alberto Antonio Rasia-Filho, and Paulo Ivo Homem de Bittencourt. "Suppressed Anti-Inflammatory Heat Shock Response in High-Risk COVID-19 Patients: Lessons from Basic Research (Inclusive Bats), Light on Conceivable Therapies." *Clinical Science* 134, no. 15 (2020): 1991–2017.

Keller, Tiffany. "150 Nonreleasable Bats Are the Legacy of One BCI Member's Chance Encounter with an Injured Bat." *Bats Magazine* 17, no. 2 (1999).

Noble, Earl G., Kevin J. Milne, and C. W. James Melling. "Heat Shock Proteins and Exercise: A Primer." *Applied Physiology, Nutrition, and Metabolism* 33, no. 5 (2008): 1050–65.

Pinar, Ortan, Yildirim Akan Ozden, Erkizan Omur, and Gedizlioglu Muhtesem. "Heat Shock Proteins in Multiple Sclerosis." *Advances in Experimental Medicine and Biology* 958 (2017): 29–42.

Salway, Kurtis D., Emily J. Gallagher, Melissa M. Page, and Jeffrey A. Stuart. "Higher Levels of Heat Shock Proteins in Longer-Lived Mammals and Birds." *Mechanism of Ageing and Development* 132, no. 6-7 (2011): 287–97.

Sørensen, Jesper Givskov, Torsten Nygaard Kristensen, and Volker Loeschcke. "The Evolutionary and Ecological Role of Heat Shock Proteins." *Ecology Letters* 6, no. 11 (2003): 1025–37.

Steelman, Andrew J. "Infection as an Environmental Trigger of Multiple Sclerosis Disease Exacerbation." *Frontiers in Immunology* 6, no. 520 (2015).

Turturici, Giuseppina, et al. "Positive or Negative Involvement of Heat Shock Proteins in Multiple Sclerosis Pathogenesis: An Overview." *Journal of Neuropathology & Experimental Neurology* 73, no. 12 (2014): 1092–1106,

Watanabe, Myrna E. "Generating Heat: New Twists in the Evolution of Endothermy." *BioScience* 55, no. 6 (2005): 470–75.

Whitham, Martin, and Matthew Benjamin Fortes. "Heat Shock Protein 72: Release and Biological Significance during Exercise." *Frontiers in Bioscience* 13 (2008): 1328–39.

Zulkifli, Idrus, et al. "A Note on Heat Shock Protein 70 Expression in Goats Subjected to Road Transportation under Hot, Humid Tropical Conditions." *Animal: An International Journal of Animal Bioscience* 4, no. 6 (2010): 973–76.

CHAPTER 10: THE EXERCISE DIET

Esser, Karyn A. Interview by author. January 27, 2022.

Kohrt, Wendy. Interview by author. January 26, 2022.

Neufer, Darrell P. Interview by author. October 26, 2016 and August 3, 2021.

Index